MOM'S GUIDE TO
DIASTASIS RECTI

MOM'S GUIDE TO DIASTASIS RECTI

A Program for Preventing and Healing Abdominal Separation Caused by Pregnancy

PAMELA ELLGEN

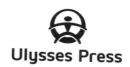

Ulysses Press

Published in the United States by:
Ulysses Press
P.O. Box 3440
Berkeley, CA 94703
www.ulyssespress.com

ISBN: 978-1-61243-661-6
Library of Congress Control Number 2016957527

Printed in the United States by United Graphics Inc.
10 9 8 7 6 5 4 3 2 1

Acquisitions: Casie Vogel
Managing editor: Claire Chun
Editor: Shayna Keyles
Proofreaders: Renee Rutledge, Lily Chou
Indexer: Sayre Van Young
Front cover design: Rebecca Lown
Interior design: what!design @ whatweb.com
Cover photos: © Rich Ellgen except mother and child © Evgeny Bakharev/shutterstock.com
Interior photos: Rich Ellgen
Models: Pamela Ellgen, Meagan Stirling

Distributed by Publishers Group West

PLEASE NOTE: This book has been written and published strictly for informational purposes, and in no way should it be used as a substitute for consultation with health care professionals. You shouldn't consider educational material herein to be the practice of medicine or to replace consultation with a physician or other medical practitioner. The author and publisher are providing you with information in this work so that you can have the knowledge and can choose, at your own risk, to act on that knowledge. The author and publisher also urge all readers to be aware of their health status and to consult health care professionals before beginning any health program.

CONTENTS

Quick-Start Guide 1

Introduction 3

Part 1: DIASTASIS RECTI 101 7
What Is Diastasis Recti? 8

Part 2: PREVENTION 21
Prevention During Pregnancy 22

Marching 24	Overhead Squat.............. 36
Side Toe Touch & Arm Raise 25	Walking Lunge............... 37
High Knee Lift.................. 26	Static Lunge 39
Front Kick & Punch.............. 27	Side Lunge 40
Frontal Deltoid Raise 28	Dead Lift................ 41
Lateral Deltoid Raise 29	Shoulder Stretch 42
Biceps Curl.................. 30	Triceps Stretch............ 43
Hammer Curl................. 31	Quadriceps Stretch........... 44
Triceps Dip.................. 32	Psoas Lunge Stretch........... 45
Lat Row.................. 33	Hamstrings Stretch 46
Squat 34	

Postpartum Prevention 47

Diaphragmatic Breathing.............. 48	Abdominal Contraction 50
Pelvic Tilt & Contraction............ 49	Kegels 51

Part 3: TREATMENT 52

Treatment Overview 53

Phase One—Activate 56

Supine Thigh Adductor 57
Glute Bridge 58
Cat Pose 59
Goblet Squat 60
Wall Plank 61
Kneeling Hay Baler 62
Crunch 63
Supine Alternating Bent-Knee Lift 64

Phase Two—Balance 65

Side-Lying Clamshell 66
Glute Bridge with Leg Extension 67
Extended Cat Pose 68
Overhead Squat 69
Walking Lunge with Chop 70
Dead Bug 71
Kneeling Psoas Stretch 72
Modified Plank 73
Reverse Crunch 74
Oblique Twist 75
Modified Side Plank 76

Phase Three—Strengthen 77

Push-Up 79
Concentration Curl 80
Arnold Press 81
Wall Squat 82
Stability Ball Bridge & Curl 83
Plank 84
Side Plank 85
Alternating Straight-Leg Lift 86
Reverse Oblique Twist 87
Stability Ball Leg Lift 88

Weight Loss 89

Marching 98
Shallow Squat 99
Side-to-Side Toe Touch 100
High Knee Lift 101
Mountain Climber 102
Jumping Jack 103
Burpee 104
Side Skate 106
Squat Jump 107
Calf Stretch 108
Kneeling Wall Stretch 108
Runner's Pose 109
Hip Stretch 109

References 110

Index 115

Acknowledgments 119

About the Author 121

QUICK-START GUIDE

If you prefer to skip over the research and jump straight to the exercises, I understand. If you've already given birth, chances are every minute is precious. Here's what you need to know to get the most out of this book:

- If you're still pregnant, turn to page 22 for a safe but challenging Prevention During Pregnancy program to increase your overall fitness and reduce the risk of diastasis recti by as much as 35 percent.

- If you've just had your baby, turn to page 47 for four postpartum exercises you can do in the hospital that have been shown to reduce diastasis recti.

- For a treatment overview, turn to page 53. Whether your baby was born six weeks ago or six years ago, this three-phase progressive program will help you reduce diastasis recti, improve core strength, and achieve a flat stomach.

Of course, always consult with your doctor before beginning any exercise routine, especially if you have or have had complications in pregnancy or delivery, particularly cesarean deliveries.

INTRODUCTION

Shortly after I gave birth to my second son by emergency cesarean section, I snuck away from home to get a pedicure. As my feet soaked in the spa tub, the nail technician asked the question every postpartum woman dreads: When are you due?

"Two weeks ago," I said.

"Wow, you look amazing," she said, thinking I was two weeks overdue.

There was an uncomfortable silence in the nail salon. I just laughed.

My body had done something amazing—it had nourished and supported a new life for nine months. Not only had it done what it was supposed to, but it also looked exactly the way it was supposed to after such an accomplishment.

I've never viewed my body with as much acceptance as I did after giving birth, even though neither birth went as I anticipated. Perhaps it was because I finally had an excuse not to have a perfect body, whatever that means. Perhaps it was because I was too smitten with my newborn to care. And perhaps it was because I had a profound new respect for my body and what it was capable of. It was empowering.

This might sound like a strange way to introduce a book about altering the physical effects of pregnancy. However, I believe physical fitness and good nutrition should always emerge from a place of self-acceptance and kindness. You have to treat your body—especially your pregnant and postpartum body—with a lot of love and respect. This means not pushing yourself to the point of injury, making sure you get enough sleep (or as much as your new baby allows), eating nourishing foods, and choosing healthy and strong over skinny.

"Exercise and eat well because you love your
body, not because you hate it."

This book is designed to help you develop healthy movement patterns during and after pregnancy so that you can handle the physical demands of caring for a newborn without pain and help your body recover from the physical effects of pregnancy. It will help you prevent and heal diastasis recti, restore pelvic floor strength, and improve core stability and strength. It will also help you reshape your waistline and reduce excess body fat in a safe and sustainable way.

Part 1 of the book explains the causes and symptoms of diastasis recti and how you can test for the condition safely in your own home. It also covers the risk factors for developing the condition, and whether or not having it predisposes you to other conditions. It explores how to prevent diastasis recti during pregnancy and the immediate postpartum period, and covers the various treatment methods available. Part 1 also discusses the other causes of stomach protrusion that affect most postpartum women.

Part 2 of the book is devoted to specific exercises for preventing diastasis recti during and immediately following pregnancy, and includes a complete pregnancy workout and exercises you can do in the hospital immediately after birth to begin healing diastasis.

Part 3, the largest section of the book, is dedicated to healing diastasis recti both for women who are newly postpartum and those who are addressing their diastasis years after childbirth. The exercises are divided into three phases to ensure safe, gradual progression. It also includes a chapter devoted to overall weight loss to reveal the strong, shapely abdominal muscles you'll develop.

The methods described in this book are backed up by the latest scientific research into diastasis recti. They're designed for busy moms to complete in just 10 minutes a day with minimal equipment and easy-to-understand exercise descriptions. Whatever your fitness level, this book will help you heal diastasis recti and improve the appearance of your waist.

MY STORY

Before I became pregnant with my first son, I exercised religiously and carefully tracked calories. Fitness was my passion, sometimes even my obsession. After several months of trying to conceive, I considered whether my low body weight and low energy intake were hindering my efforts to get pregnant. (You think?) So I relaxed my attitude toward food, slowed down the intense workouts, and gained a few pounds.

Within a month or two, I got pregnant. For some reason, I threw all caution to the wind regarding nutrition and exercise. I stopped working out and my grocery budget burgeoned, along with my waistline. I enjoyed milkshakes and burgers after every doctor's appointment—yes, even when they came weekly. By the time I was 25 weeks pregnant, people were asking whether I was having triplets and thought I might go into labor at any minute. Not funny.

During my third trimester, a distant cousin with four of her own children cautioned me about diastasis recti. She said I shouldn't use my abdominal muscles at all after birth to avoid irreversible abdominal separation. Yikes! She put the fear of diastasis in me, and I vowed to brace when coughing or sneezing and used triceps pushup to get out of bed so as not to engage my abs at all.

My water broke the day after my due date and I labored for an intense 24 hours without much progress before being wheeled into the operating room for a C-section. As far as I was concerned, delivering a healthy baby was all that mattered, so I was overjoyed to welcome my son into the world however he came. I left the hospital a few days later with a stack of maxi pads, enormous mesh panties, a painful incision, and an extra 40 pounds.

About a pound of weight a day came off the first two weeks, giving me incredible hope for hopping into my pre-pregnancy jeans within a few months. But, eventually, it stalled, and I began the long road to regaining the strength, endurance, and shape I had before pregnancy. Through consistent exercise and sound nutrition, a year later I was back to my pre-pregnancy weight and had built back most of the muscle I had lost.

However, I was still hesitant about doing abdominal exercises. Sometimes I felt a strange tinge of pain at the site of my incision, and I always noticed "doming" in my stomach when I did crunches. "Six-pack abs are made in the kitchen, not the gym," I told myself. So, I didn't invest much time in ab exercises.

When my son was two years old, I became a certified personal trainer with the National Academy of Sports Medicine (NASM). It had a profound impact on the way I approached fitness and gave me an insatiable hunger for reading studies on fitness and nutrition in medical journals. Shortly thereafter, I began training clients at a local gym and writing about health and fitness for LIVESTRONG and eventually Spinning.com, Jillian Michaels, and the *Huffington Post*.

I became pregnant with my second son when my first was three years old, and I committed to doing things differently this time around. I continued running and weight lifting, began practicing yoga more consistently, and enrolled in the NASM training course for prenatal fitness.

Two days before my due date, I participated in a live seminar to renew my training credentials. It involved a weekend full of intense workouts, including resistance training, core exercise, and plyometric jumps. Because of the fitness level I had maintained during pregnancy, it was easy (although the instructor did look at me sideways more than once while I was executing 180-degree turn and squat jumps).

This time, I had a scheduled C-section and began postpartum exercise as soon as I was capable of standing. It involved gentle walking around the hospital ward. It felt good to move and this immediately improved my blood flow, oxygen levels, and general outlook.

I left the hospital in my yoga pants with about 20 extra pounds. Recovery was much easier the second time around, and I gradually worked toward the fitness level I had at the end of my pregnancy, taking care not to do anything that put stress on the surgical incision. The weight melted off and within three weeks, I was happily wearing some of my pre-pregnancy clothes, although it took several more months to really return to my pre-pregnancy shape.

Through all this time, my wariness about abdominal exercises remained. My core strength was unimpressive. And it showed. I constantly had a protruding belly, even years after my son was born. Even when I was the same weight as before pregnancy, it stuck out. Part of the problem was poor postural habits picked up during adolescent growth spurts and pregnancy. Some of it was digestive. (Going gluten-free helped.) But, ultimately, I had to address the most obvious reason for my protruding belly: weak abdominal muscles.

When I began researching for this book, I heard the familiar refrain by diastasis recti experts: don't do crunches—they'll make it worse! They advocated splints, alignment techniques, and thousands of repetitions of exercises that targeted certain abdominal muscles while attempting to avoid activating others. If you didn't follow the programs to the letter, they wouldn't work.

In the end, it was the established and emerging scientific research on diastasis recti that set the record straight: progressive abdominal exercises that bring the rectus abdominis muscles together without producing "doming" can reduce diastasis recti. Study after study finds that crunches result in decreased distance between the rectus abdominis muscles, whereas the drawing-in maneuver (the exercise advocated by many popular programs for diastasis recti) actually increases this distance during exercise. This research laid the groundwork for the program in this book. Through it, I learned how to scale abdominal exercises to my fitness level, to avoid doming and pain at the incision site, and to bring the rectus abdominis together. The exercises helped me shrink my diastasis in half, regain core strength, shape defined abdominal muscles, and flatten my stomach for good. And I know they will for you, too!

Part 1

DIASTASIS RECTI 101

WHAT IS DIASTASIS RECTI?

Diastasis recti is a stretching and widening of the linea alba, which is the connective tissue that runs down the center of your abdomen and connects the major abdominal muscles: the external obliques, internal obliques, transversus abdominis, and rectus abdominis. Your abdominal muscles work together to flex and twist your trunk, and to maintain proper posture.

LINEA ALBA: located along the center of the abdomen from the sternum to the pubic symphysis.

EXTERNAL OBLIQUES: located on the sides and front of the abdomen. Responsible for trunk lateral flexion and rotation.

INTERNAL OBLIQUES: located beneath the external obliques. Responsible for trunk lateral flexion and rotation. Aids in respiration.

TRANSVERSUS ABDOMINIS: located deepest within the abdomen, beneath the internal obliques. Responsible for pulling the abdominal wall inward to increase intra-abdominal pressure.

RECTUS ABDOMINIS: located on the front of the abdomen, divided into two "halves." Responsible for trunk flexion and posterior pelvic tilt.

Everyone has a natural gap between the right and left halves of their rectus abdominis—you can see it in people with exceptional ab definition. This gap is considered a diastasis when the connective tissue stretches to be larger than normal. So, what's normal? The official diagnostic criteria for diastasis recti varies among medical professionals, perhaps in part because there's natural variation in the width of linea alba between individuals. The most common definition is that a diastasis recti is a width greater than 2.7 centimeters, or about two finger widths. Measurements are

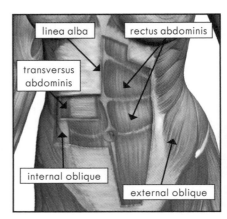

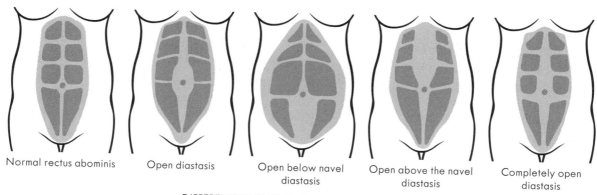

| Normal rectus abominis | Open diastasis | Open below navel diastasis | Open above the navel diastasis | Completely open diastasis |

DIFFERENT VARIATIONS OF DIASTASIS RECTI

typically taken above and below the navel while lying down and lifting the head and sometimes shoulders off the floor.

Diastasis recti doesn't hurt the way a pulled muscle does because the linea alba is fibrous, composed mostly of collagen, and contains virtually no nerves or blood vessels. Diastasis recti can occur above the navel, below the navel, or in both places at once. Interestingly, the site of the diastasis doesn't always correspond to the site of abdominal protrusion, according to research published in the *Journal of Plastic and Reconstructive Surgery*.

It has been said that "what gets measured gets managed," and diastasis recti, like your body weight, can easily be measured. Place your fingers into the gap caused by diastasis and you can determine, with relative accuracy, how wide it is. From there you can go about reducing it through interventions such as exercise, physical therapy, and support belts. The problem is that, like your weight, the size of the diastasis only tells part of the story, and shrinking it may or may not give you the slender stomach you want.

Wait, what? You're probably thinking, "I thought this was a book on preventing and healing diastasis recti!" It is, don't worry. But it's about more than that. It's also about strengthening pelvic floor muscles, enhancing spinal stability, and improving core strength, as well as reducing abdominal fat. All of these are essential elements in shaping a defined stomach. And that's what this book is about.

CAUSES

Diastasis recti is caused by excess intra-abdominal pressure, pregnancy being the most obvious and common cause of the condition. During pregnancy, your growing baby and expanding uterus cause the abdominal muscles and connective tissue to stretch, aided in part by the hormones estrogen and relaxin. This process is healthy and natural; virtually all pregnant women have some degree of abdominal separation and thinning of the linea alba during and immediately following pregnancy. In most women, especially those who didn't remain physically active during pregnancy, the rectus abdominis muscle is also weak and overstretched.

While diastasis recti has been linked to pregnancy weight gain, advanced maternal age, or giving birth to large-birth-weight babies, a study published in 2015 in the journal *Manual Therapy* found no such correlation. For about 35 to 40 percent of women, diastasis occurred at six months postpartum, regardless of those factors.

Diastasis can also occur due to improper weightlifting technique, excessive or poorly executed abdominal exercises, and even belly fat itself. Hence, both men and women can have the condition. It can also occur in newborns, especially premature babies, when the rectus abdominis hasn't fully developed and isn't fused at the midline.

SYMPTOMS

Quite often, the perceived symptoms of diastasis recti are actually symptoms of weak, overstretched abdominal muscles. And many cases of diastasis recti are asymptomatic. Here are two of the primary symptoms attributed to diastasis recti, although they may or may not be caused by the condition.

REDUCED ABDOMINAL STRENGTH

Diastasis recti is correlated with reduced abdominal strength. A study published in the *Journal of Orthopaedic & Sports Physical Therapy* observed this effect in 40 postpartum women aged 25 to 37. Researchers measured trunk flexion, rotation strength, and endurance. They found that during the approximately six-month postpartum period when the gap caused by diastasis recti naturally decreased, abdominal strength increased. It's unclear from these results whether the increased abdominal strength contributed to the reduced diastasis or the other way around; a better way of thinking about it is that overstretched abdominal muscles and an overstretched linea alba contribute to reduced abdominal strength.

ABDOMINAL PROTRUSION

Diastasis recti may or may not cause abdominal protrusion, as evidenced by a study published in the journal *Plastic and Reconstructive Surgery*. In the study, 92 abdominoplasty patients volunteered for measurements of the linea alba to be taken during surgery. Researchers noted the linea alba had a limited range of stretch, usually between 1 and 2 inches, and this had no correlation to the size of their abdominal protrusion. They concluded "abdominal wall protrusions are caused by the stretching of the entire abdominal wall and not only the linea alba. Thus, significant abdominal wall protrusions may occur without diastasis and flat abdomens may exhibit a diastasis."

Based on these studies, we can say that the presence of diastasis recti doesn't sentence you to a protruding belly. And, unfortunately, healing it won't guarantee you a flat stomach. The idea that it could makes a fine selling point for diastasis recti programs, but this isn't necessarily supported by science. Instead, a comprehensive approach to strengthening the core muscles—which, if done properly, can heal diastasis—will correct abdominal protrusion.

HOW TO CHECK FOR DIASTASIS RECTI

Before you test for diastasis recti, remember that home tests aren't an exact science. Pelvic tilt, co-contraction of the transversus abdominis, and the degree of abdominal contraction when you're taking measurements will affect the width and depth of the diastasis. With this test, you'll be assessing the degree of your own diastasis and how it changes over time.

1. Lie on your back on a mat, with knees bent and feet flat on the ground.

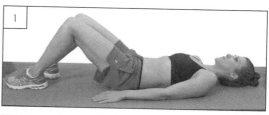

2. With one arm stretched toward your pelvis, fingers pointed down and palm facing toward your face, lower your fingers toward your belly button.

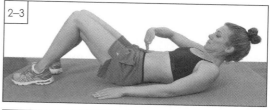

3. Raise your head and shoulders off of the floor just enough to engage your abdominal muscles.

4. Lower your fingers into the space between the two sides of your abdominal muscles.

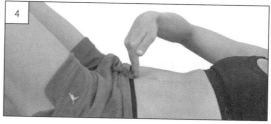

5. Measure about two inches above your belly button, and again two inches below your belly button.

Measure the width and depth of separation. Note your results. A moderate diastasis is two fingers wide or greater, and about one to two centimeters deep. Any distance greater than this should be evaluated by your physician.

In a clinical setting, diastasis may be measured using calipers, which are more precise than finger-width measurements and are used in most of the research cited throughout this book.

Ultrasound imaging is another method of testing. When performed by a knowledgeable and trained practitioner, it can be an effective measure of inter-rectus distance (the distance between the halves of the rectus abdominis) and used again to determine the effectiveness of treatment.

RISKS

Although many conditions can occur simultaneously with diastasis recti, such as pelvic floor disorders, low back pain, and hernia, there isn't a medical consensus on whether the condition itself is harmful to women's function. I spoke to one researcher who was hesitant to even assess the effects of diastasis recti in future research because she could find no definitive evidence that it compromised women's function.

PELVIC FLOOR DISORDERS

Following pregnancy, many women have pelvic floor weakness, urinary incontinence, and occasionally even pelvic organ prolapse. However, it's important to note that none of these conditions is caused by diastasis recti, despite what popular exercise regimens for the condition advertise. In fact, a study published by Norwegian researchers in 2016 found that diastasis recti seems to occur less often in women who've reduced vaginal resting pressure, reduced pelvic floor muscle strength, urinary incontinence, and pelvic organ prolapse. They found that women with diastasis recti at 21 weeks pregnant had greater vaginal resting pressure, strength, and endurance than women without the separation. Moreover, following pregnancy, women with diastasis were 10 percent less likely to have pelvic organ prolapse.

LOW BACK PAIN

Diastasis recti is also often associated with low back pain. However, a study published in the journal *Manual Therapy* in 2015 found no correlation between incidence of lumbo-pelvic pain and diastasis recti at six months after pregnancy. The story may be different when the diastasis is accompanied by a ventral (abdominal) hernia, though, as another study published in the journal *Hernia* in 2015 found that surgery to correct severe diastasis recti and concurrent midline hernias significantly improved low back pain. However, it's unlikely that diastasis itself causes low back pain; weak core muscles and incorrect posture do.

VENTRAL HERNIA

In rare cases, diastasis recti can result in an abdominal hernia, which is when tissue from the abdomen pushes through weaker tissue. Symptoms of a hernia include a bulge or lump in the abdomen, pain, nausea, and vomiting, although some hernias don't present symptoms. Hernias are associated with previous abdominal surgery, including cesarean section. About 2 out of every 1,000 women will require surgery to correct an incisional hernia following a C-section. If you suspect you have an abdominal hernia, see your doctor before proceeding with the exercises in this book.

PREVENTION & TREATMENT

Thinning and stretching of the linea alba and rectus abdominis is one of many ways our bodies are designed to handle pregnancy and childbirth. Some degree of diastasis during these periods is healthy and natural, although women with greater abdominal strength before pregnancy will experience a lesser degree of abdominal separation. Exercise is the only proven method of prevention against diastasis recti during pregnancy.

Researchers have observed that diastasis recti heals the most quickly during the first eight weeks following pregnancy and then plateaus without further intervention, although a study published in the *Journal of Orthopaedic & Sports Physical Therapy* found further, albeit small, reductions in diastasis recti between seven weeks and six months postpartum.

After pregnancy, treatment methods include targeted abdominal exercise, support belts, and surgery, and each of these methods has varying degrees of efficacy.

PRENATAL EXERCISE

Exercise during pregnancy can reduce the prevalence of diastasis recti by 35 percent, according to a 2014 review published in *Physiotherapy*. Prenatal exercise has several other positive outcomes as well, including reduced maternal weight gain, hypertension, and gestational diabetes, as well as improved feelings of well-being, lower incidence of pregnancy-related pain and discomfort, and better sleep. Both aerobic and resistance exercise have been shown to be safe and effective during pregnancy.

This book includes a full-body prenatal workout that can be scaled to your fitness level. However, virtually any physical activity without inherent risk of falling or injury is safe during pregnancy. If you did it before pregnancy, you can likely continue it throughout your pregnancy. Of course, always check with your doctor before you engage in any exercise program, especially if you have any pregnancy complications.

POSTPARTUM EXERCISE & GENERAL MOVEMENT

Conventional wisdom on postpartum exercise advises women to wait six weeks after childbirth to resume a regular exercise routine. However, the American College of Obstetrics and Gynecology says physical activity can be resumed as soon as it's physically and medically safe, which will vary from one woman to another. Some are capable of engaging in an exercise routine within days of delivery. The organization also noted that there's no credible evidence to indicate that, in the absence of medical complications, resuming physical activity soon after pregnancy will result in adverse effects.

One of the primary benefits of postpartum exercise, particularly strength training, is that it can help you improve spinal stability and develop proper lifting techniques, both of which can help you avoid worsening your diastasis recti. The exercises in this book, both in the prenatal workout and in the three phases of the postpartum program, are designed to help you develop proper lifting technique.

Ultimately, listen to your doctor and to your own body, not arbitrary rules about what you should and shouldn't be capable of after your pregnancy.

However, there are some activities that can put tension on the linea alba following pregnancy. Exercises that require spinal extension, including back bends and the yoga poses cobra and upward dog, should be avoided when recovering from diastasis recti. The same applies to weighted twisting maneuvers, such as the Russian Twist. Additionally, improper lifting techniques, especially when carrying heavy objects such as car seats, can contribute to increased intra-abdominal pressure and place tension on the linea alba, which can worsen diastasis recti. If you practice child-wearing, placing the child on your back creates the least amount of intra-abdominal pressure, especially when walking and as walking speed is increased.

POSTURE

Throughout the following chapters, I refer to the "braced neutral spine position." I learned this term and the technique for achieving it from Dr. Kelly Starrett, author of the book *Becoming a Supple Leopard*. He says braced neutral spine is "the most utilitarian position for the spine because it allows you to handle load safely and transmit force efficiently. For the majority of movements, you don't want your spine to deviate from this neutral position."

Braced neutral spine is proper posture, but not in the way we typically think of it (i.e., an arched lower back, drawn in stomach, retracted shoulders, and puffed chest). Instead, it involves firming the thighs and buttocks, contracting the abdominal muscles, stacking the ribs over the hips and pelvis, and lifting through the crown of your head.

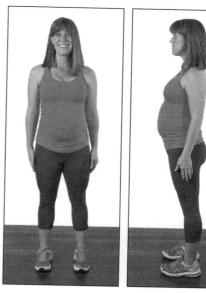

Braced neutral spine

If you take away nothing else from this book, learning how to stay in braced neutral spine position throughout your day, especially when lifting, will reduce your risk of injury, improve core stability, and improve the appearance of your stomach. More importantly to the aim of this book, it will reduce tension placed on connective tissue and train you to use your bones and muscles to support your weight. Braced neutral spine (page 54) is the first exercise taught in the Treatment Overview.

ABDOMINAL EXERCISE

Popular advice on diastasis recti cautions women to avoid any abdominal flexion (e.g., crunches) for as long as a diastasis persists, in fear of worsening it. Instead, women are encouraged to perform exercises designed to activate the transverse abdominis muscle, particularly the "drawing-in" maneuver, which involves pulling the navel toward the spine. It's also called abdominal "hollowing" and, according to this theory, should be practiced both in static positions and in general while engaging in other activities. There are a few problems with this approach.

First, it's difficult, if not impossible, to fully isolate any muscle during movement or isometric contraction; synergist (helping) and antagonist (resisting) muscles will be activated to some degree, which is essential to how your body functions as a system.

What Is Diastasis Recti?   15

Second, the drawing-in maneuver doesn't increase spinal stability, which is especially important for pregnant and postpartum women. Spinal stability is already compromised during pregnancy due to the increased load of the baby, decreased strength of the abdominal muscles, and an anterior pelvic tilt. A study published in the *Archives of Physical Medicine and Rehabilitation* in 2007 found that, compared with full abdominal muscle contraction (activities that use all abdominal muscles), the abdominal hollowing technique provided 32 percent less spinal stability. The authors concluded, "There seems to be no mechanical rationale for using an abdominal hollow, or the transversus abdominis, to enhance stability. Bracing creates patterns that better enhance stability." Therefore, techniques that encourage activation of all abdominal muscles, not just the transversus abdominis, are more useful for enhancing spinal stability and improving movement patterns for new moms.

Finally, and perhaps most relevant to this book, by using the drawing-in maneuver, inter-rectus distance actually increases. Yes, you read that correctly. The exercise touted as the most effective treatment for diastasis actually widens the gap, at least during the exercise. A study published in 2015 in the journal *Physiotherapy* found that inter-rectus distance below the navel was significantly greater during drawing-in exercises compared with at rest. The authors noted, "… the muscle bellies and abdominal fascia are moved apart, which may reduce the ability of the muscles to generate enough tensile force." That's particularly concerning for women who've had a C-section, because the point of measurement was below the navel.

Conversely, they found that inter-rectus distance was significantly reduced during abdominal crunch exercises compared with at rest. (Finally, some vindication for crunches!) Several other studies have observed similar effects, and these are included in the references section of this book.

Research conducted on the long-term effects of abdominal exercise on diastasis recti shows significant positive results. There are only a handful of studies on exercise and diastasis, which makes any firm conclusions difficult to establish with absolute certainty. However, because our goal isn't simply to narrow the diastasis but to increase core strength and spinal stability, develop healthy movement patterns, and improve the appearance of our stomachs, the availability of quality research is virtually infinite. Here are a few more examples.

A study published in the *Journal of Obstetrics and Gynecology* evaluated 50 postpartum women who had given birth vaginally and had a 3-centimeter diastasis. The study found that women who engaged in two therapeutic exercise interventions immediately following childbirth (one was given 6 hours following birth, a second 18 hours following) had more than twice the reduction in diastasis recti than the control group. The therapy consisted of five simple exercises designed to activate the abdominal muscles and pelvic floor, including crunches. Assessments were taken at these intervals as well. Women who received the therapy had a 12.5 percent reduction in diastasis over the course of treatment, compared to a 5.4 percent reduction in the control group.

Another study published by the World Academy of Science, Engineering, and Technology (WASET) compared the effectiveness of long-term targeted abdominal exercise to the effectiveness of wearing an abdominal support belt. Scientists divided women into two groups and observed them from the second day after delivery until six weeks after birth. The first group used an abdominal support belt every day during that period. The second group engaged in monitored 30-minute abdominal exercise sessions three times each week, and repeated the program at home on the other days. The exercises, which included crunches, were designed to activate and strengthen the abdominal and pelvic floor muscles.

Not surprisingly, the second group saw significant increases in abdominal muscle strength and had a pronounced reduction in waist-to-hip ratio and diastasis recti compared to the first group. Researchers noted that strengthening the abdominal muscles in this manner is both safe and effective, and stated, "It's important to begin postnatal abdominal exercises that are graded to the rate of recovery and the pre-delivery level of fitness." In light of the evidence presented in this and other studies, I fully agree with this approach.

However, people with diastasis recti should avoid "doming" during abdominal exercise, which is when the lower abdomen pushes upward during the contraction phase of the movement. If this occurs, simply regress the exercise so that you can complete it without doming. For example, if Alternating Straight-Leg Lifts (page 86) produce doming, regress the move to Supine Alternating Bent-Knee Lifts (page 64). I designed this program to progress gradually through three phases, but each person will have her own limitations. You should always listen to your own body.

POSTPARTUM SUPPORT BELT

Many hospitals provide elastic support belts for women following childbirth, specifically after cesarean section. They can also be purchased online or through your obstetrician. The bands are designed to promote spinal alignment, provide support for weakened abdominal muscles, and take the pressure off a cesarean incision.

They're also used to treat diastasis recti. In the WASET study referenced above, the research subjects who wore a support belt daily over the course of the six-week study saw a five percent reduction in diastasis recti. However, no control group was included in the study, making it impossible to know whether the diastasis would've closed naturally (as it usually does during this period) or perhaps even more quickly without a belt.

The prevailing theory behind abdominal support belts to treat diastasis recti is that they relieve tension on the linea alba. One popular program sells a band that "takes the 'stretch' off of the overstretched tissue, making it narrower." This theory has numerous problems, not the least of which is that the "stretch" has already been alleviated—your growing uterus is no longer pushing against your abdomen. A study published in the journal *PLoS One* in 2014 confirmed this, concluding that intra-abdominal pressure significantly decreases to normal values after delivery.

The theory also assumes that physical tissue has similar properties to elastic, which it doesn't. To show the fallacy of that logic, imagine a headband stretched around a beach ball and left for several weeks. When you remove the band, it would be overstretched and wouldn't fit snuggly on your head. Refraining from wearing it on your head wouldn't spare the headband from further stretching or undo the initial stretch. Additionally, there isn't enough compelling evidence about whether physical tissue responds to compression by returning to its original size.

Ultimately, if you find a support belt comfortable and flattering and it encourages better posture and movement patterns, wear it for a while. However, long-term use doesn't have any proven benefits, so don't expect it to shrink your diastasis or train your abs for you.

NUTRITION

There's no peer-reviewed research on the effects of sound nutrition during or after pregnancy on diastasis recti. Popular advice to drink bone broth or take collagen supplements is purely speculative. It probably won't hurt you, but there's no scientific evidence to support its use for reducing diastasis recti.

However, this book is about more than simply shrinking diastasis recti. It's about eliminating belly protrusion, and good nutrition is an essential step toward this goal. See page 89 for a thorough discussion of nutrition for weight loss.

SURGERY

Surgery is considered a last resort for fixing diastasis recti, but it may be especially helpful when the diastasis is accompanied by a ventral hernia. Prosthetic mesh is sometimes used in surgery, and a 2015 retrospective review published in the journal *Plastic and Reconstructive*

Surgery found that mesh repair was both safe and durable. For less severe diastasis recti, when there's no loose skin, a minimally invasive endoscopic procedure can fix the separation. If you believe surgery is the best option for you, see a board-certified plastic surgeon for a complete evaluation and discuss your options.

OTHER CAUSES OF BELLY PROTRUSION

Diastasis recti isn't the sole cause of post-pregnancy belly protrusion. A few other conditions are likely culprits, particularly in postpartum women.

ANTERIOR PELVIC TILT

When the top of your pelvis rotates forward, you develop a pronounced arch in your lower back and your stomach and buttocks protrude. If you're having trouble visualizing it, just think of virtually every fitness inspiration picture you've seen on Pinterest. Women often arch their backs, extend their abdomen to make it appear flatter, and stick out their butts. When people are in this pose, you'll notice that the waistband of their workout shorts descends in the front and is higher in the back.

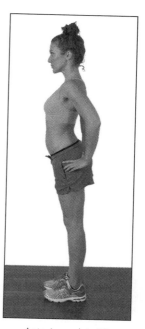

Anterior pelvic tilt is common among pregnant women to compensate for the weight of the growing baby. It's easier to rest on the connective tissue of the abdomen (which worsens diastasis recti) than to maintain erect posture by activating the core muscles. Anterior pelvic tilt can persist after pregnancy and may be a significant cause of belly protrusion—it certainly was for me. The exercises in this book are designed to simultaneously address anterior pelvic tilt and abdominal strengthening.

Anterior pelvic tilt

DIGESTIVE PROBLEMS

Food sensitivities, allergies, and celiac disease can all cause gas, bloating, constipation, and abdominal distension. If you have a known problem with certain foods, clearly you should avoid them. More likely, you're not aware of what causes your digestive discomfort. Here are a few areas to consider with your health care provider.

Foods containing wheat and dairy cause gas and bloating for some people. These foods are present in a larger class of ingredients known as fermentable oligo-, di-, monosaccharides, and polyols (FODMAPs), which are fermentable carbohydrates that support the healthy bacteria in your digestive tract. When your digestive system is imbalanced, such as in the case of small-intestinal bacterial overgrowth (SIBO), eliminating FODMAPs for a short time may provide relief. Some of the more common FODMAPs include apples, watermelon, peaches, cruciferous vegetables, onions, garlic, wheat, dairy, and some legumes. These are otherwise healthy foods, so doing a low-FODMAP diet should be a last resort when other dietary interventions have failed.

Interestingly, some of the foods on the list of FODMAPs—onions, garlic, cabbage, and broccoli—are thought to provoke gas in breastfed babies when consumed by their mothers. While I never noticed this effect in my kids, removing wheat, dairy, and soy from my diet had a profound impact on them, essentially eliminating reflux and colic.

Allergy tests, celiac screening, and a simple elimination diet can be helpful in identifying which foods might be causing you distress. Additionally, make sure you're drinking at least 96 ounces of water daily and eating fiber-rich plant foods to ensure regular elimination.

VISCERAL FAT

Unlike subcutaneous fat, which sits just below the skin, visceral fat dwells more deeply within the abdomen and surrounds the internal organs. Think "beer belly." Although visceral fat can cause or worsen diastasis recti, it gives you a round, distended stomach even without a diastasis. The effects of visceral fat are even more insidious than a bulging belly. It increases cardiovascular risk, insulin resistance, metabolic disorders, markers of inflammation, and LDL (bad) cholesterol.

Fortunately, visceral fat responds particularly well to exercise and dietary changes, even more so than subcutaneous fat does. The section on weight loss starting on page 89 is devoted to the topic of fat loss and provides nutrition and exercise strategies that will help you eliminate overall body fat and visceral fat. Most of my personal training clients come to me with the goal of fat loss, so I'm particularly excited about this chapter.

Part 2

PREVENTION

PREVENTION DURING PREGNANCY

Exercise during pregnancy has been shown to reduce the risk of developing diastasis recti. It can also reduce pregnancy-related discomfort and help you build strength for caring for your newborn. Most exercise routines that challenge your cardiovascular system and build strength and mobility will be beneficial during pregnancy. So, if you're already participating in an exercise program that you enjoy, continue with that and add the strength workout below as you feel comfortable. You may already be doing many of these moves in your training regimen.

If you were sedentary before pregnancy, add a 30-minute walk to your day, increasing speed and elevation as you're comfortable, to create a gentle cardiovascular workout. The following strength workout can be scaled to all fitness levels by increasing resistance, and includes foundational strength movements that will help you during and after pregnancy.

It's important to perform the warm-up and cool-down. Warming up slowly elevates your heart rate, increases blood flow, and improves range of motion; the cool-down stretches the muscles you worked out and gradually brings your heart rate down.

BASIC STRENGTH & FLEXIBILITY WORKOUT

	EXERCISE	DURATION
Warm-Up	Marching (page 24)	60 seconds
	Side Toe Touch & Arm Raise (page 25)	60 seconds
	High Knee Lift (page 26)	60 seconds
	Front Kick & Punch (page 27)	60 seconds
Workout	Frontal Deltoid Raise (page 28) or Lateral Deltoid Raise (page 29)	8–12 reps each arm
	Biceps Curl (page 30) or Hammer Curl (page 31)	8–12 reps each arm
	Triceps Dip (page 32)	8–12 reps
	Lat Row (page 33)	10–12 reps
	Squat (page 34) or Overhead Squat (page 36)	10–12 reps (Squat) 8 reps (Overheat Squat)
	Walking Lunge (page 37), Static Lunge (page 39), or Side Lunge (page 40)	10–12 reps each leg
	Dead Lift (page 41)	10–12 reps
Cool-Down	Shoulder Stretch (page 42)	30 seconds per arm
	Triceps Stretch (page 43)	30 seconds per arm
	Quadriceps Stretch (page 44)	30 seconds per leg
	Psoas Lunge Stretch (page 45)	30 seconds per leg
	Hamstrings Stretch (page 46)	30 seconds per leg

MARCHING

STARTING POSITION: Stand with your feet hip-width apart and your arms at your sides.

1–2. March in place, allowing your arms to swing naturally by your sides. Continue for 60 seconds.

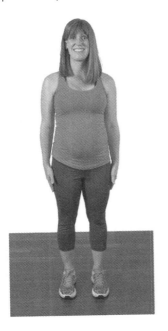

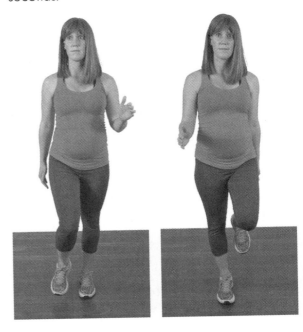

SIDE TOE TOUCH & ARM RAISE

STARTING POSITION: Stand with your feet hip-width apart and your arms at your sides.

1. While tapping one foot to the side, sweep your arms to the sides until they're extended overhead. Think jumping jacks without the jump.

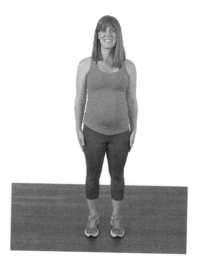

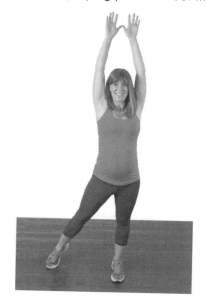

2. Lower your arms to your sides as you tap the opposite foot to the side. Repeat both steps for 60 seconds.

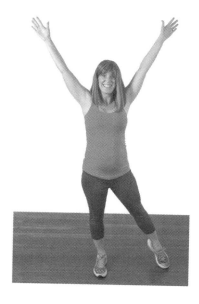

HIGH KNEE LIFT

STARTING POSITION: Stand with your feet hip-width apart and your arms at your sides.

1–2. Lift one knee until your thigh is parallel with the floor and pat it gently with your hand. Lower, and lift the other knee. Repeat for 60 seconds.

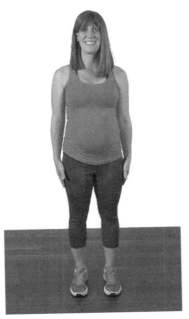

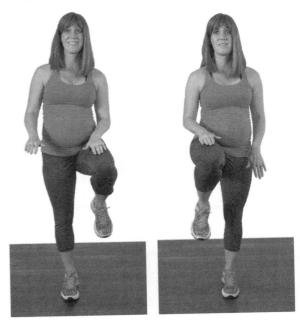

FRONT KICK & PUNCH

STARTING POSITION: Stand with your feet hip-width apart and your arms at your sides.

1–2. Kick one foot and punch with the opposite arm forward, crossing the midline of your body.

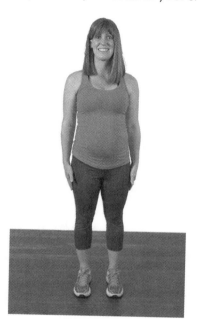

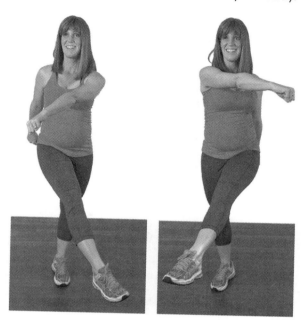

FRONTAL DELTOID RAISE

This exercise strengthens your shoulders, improves shoulder mobility, and challenges your core stabilizing muscles. Even if you're accustomed to lifting heavier weights, a light dumbbell will likely provide sufficient challenge with this exercise. This exercise and the biceps curl exercise (page 30) are done with alternating limbs to challenge and improve core stabilization. However, if you're short on time, you can perform the exercises with both arms simultaneously.

STARTING POSITION: Stand in a braced neutral position with your feet hip-width apart. Hold a light dumbbell in each hand and allow them to rest in front of your thigh, with your palms facing your body.

1. Raise one dumbbell in front of you until it's overhead, keeping your wrist neutral and your palm facing down and then forward. Keep your abdominal muscles engaged throughout the move. If you have a shorter range of motion, raise the bell until just before your shoulder feels tight.

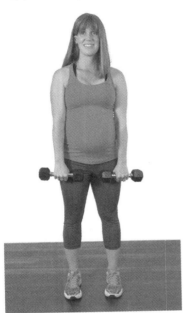

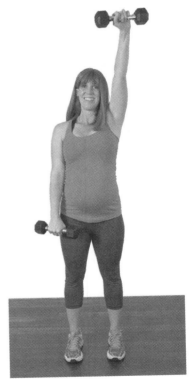

Slowly and with control, lower your arm back to starting position. Repeat on the other side.

Complete 8 to 12 repetitions.

LATERAL DELTOID RAISE

Caring for a young child involves moving and lifting in all planes of motion. Work your deltoids from a different angle by performing deltoid lifts to the sides. You can do this move with alternating arms to challenge your core stabilizing muscles, as in the previous exercise, or do both arms at the same time to finish the exercise in less time.

STARTING POSITION: Stand in a braced neutral position with your feet hip-width apart. Hold a light dumbbell in each hand and allow them to rest along your sides.

1. Raise a dumbbell to the side until your arm is nearly parallel with the floor. Don't extend beyond shoulder level.

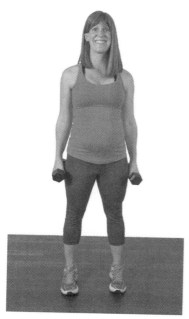

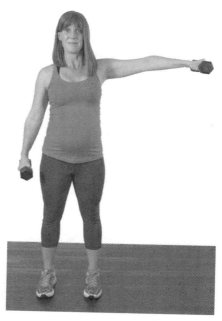

Slowly and with control, lower the dumbbell back to starting position.

Complete 8 to 12 repetitions with each arm.

BICEPS CURL

Increasing arm strength will help you carry your baby, especially when lifting and lowering her car seat.

STARTING POSITION: Stand in a braced neutral position with your feet hip-width apart. Hold a medium dumbbell in each hand and allow them to rest in front of your hips with your palms facing forward.

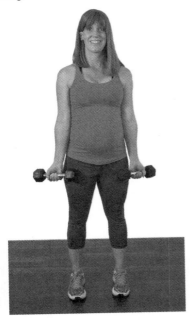

1. Bring one dumbbell up toward your chest.

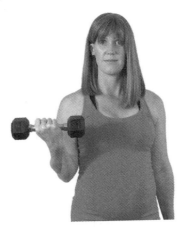

Slowly and with control, lower the dumbbell back to starting position. Repeat on the other side.

Complete 8 to 12 repetitions.

COMMON FAULTS: The dumbbell doesn't need to come all the way to your shoulder. Stop when it's just above chest level.

HAMMER CURL

Work your biceps from a different angle by performing hammer curls.

STARTING POSITION: Stand in a braced neutral position with your feet hip-width apart. Hold a medium dumbbell in each hand and allow them to rest along your sides.

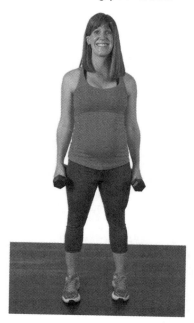

1. Bring one dumbbell up toward your shoulder so that the end of the dumbbell is facing up.

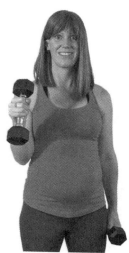

Slowly and with control, lower the dumbbell back to starting position. Repeat on the other side.

Complete 8 to 12 repetitions.

COMMON FAULTS: Don't swing the dumbbells as you complete the exercise.

TRICEPS DIP

The triceps and biceps work together in lifting maneuvers and should receive equal attention in your arm-training routine.

STARTING POSITION: Sit on the edge of a chair or bench with your hands on the edge of the bench, fingers pointed forward and down. Plant your feet about hip-width apart on the floor in front of you. Push with your hands to lift your butt off the chair so you are positioned right in front of the chair.

1. Keeping your back close to the chair and your elbows pointing straight back, bend at your shoulders and elbows to lower your butt toward the floor. Pause at the bottom of the move.

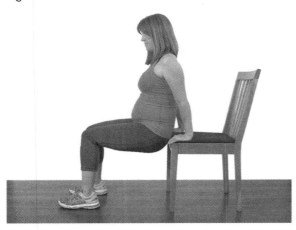

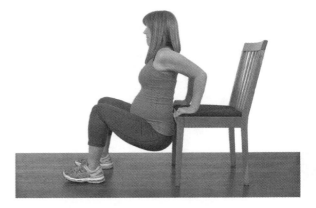

Push through your hands to rise to the starting position.

Complete 8 to 12 repetitions.

CHANGE IT UP: To make this move more difficult, extend one leg in front of you so that it's parallel with the floor throughout the move.

COMMON FAULTS: Don't allow your elbows to flare toward the sides or your hips to shift away from the bench.

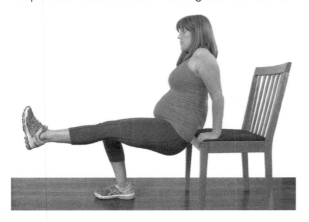

LAT ROW

Your latissimus dorsi muscle is the largest muscle in your back and an essential part of core stabilization and strength. Using this muscle in conjunction with your legs (instead of using your lower back) to lift objects from the floor will help protect your back from injury.

STARTING POSITION: Stand in a braced neutral position with your feet hip-width apart. Hinge forward from your hips and place one hand on a bench or chair. Hold a large dumbbell in the opposite hand with your palm facing the midline of your body. Continue contracting your core muscles and maintain a neutral (not rounded or arched) spine.

1. Pull the weight toward your hip, elevating your elbow behind you. Pause when the weight barely grazes your side.

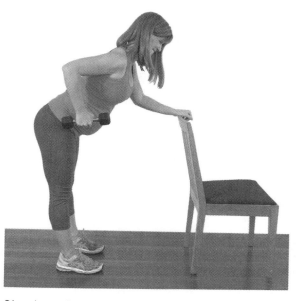

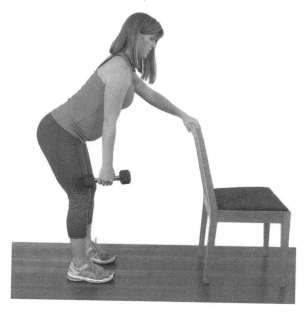

Slowly and with control, lower the weight to the starting position.

Complete 10 to 12 repetitions and then switch sides.

COMMON FAULTS: Don't rotate your spine through the move, but keep your hips and shoulders square toward the floor.

SQUAT

Properly executed squats are one of the best exercises anyone can do, especially pregnant women. They engage your core muscles, improve hip mobility, and strengthen your legs, all of which can help you avoid resting on your connective tissue during movement. If you do no other exercise in this book, do squats.

STARTING POSITION: Stand in a braced neutral position with your feet shoulder-width apart (wider is okay), knees aligned over your ankles, and toes pointing forward or barely turned out. Allow your arms to rest at your sides or extend them in front of you at shoulder level.

1. Lower your hips toward the floor as you bend your knees, allowing your upper body to hinge forward slightly. Keep your core muscles contracted and maintain a neutral (not rounded or arched) spine. Pause at the bottom of the move.

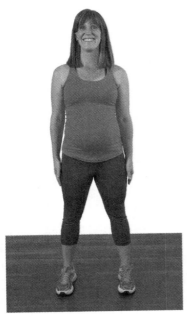

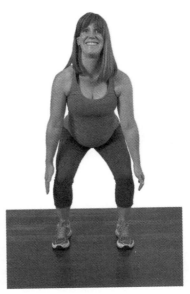

Press through your heels as you straighten your legs and rise to the starting position. Contract your gluteal muscles at the top of the move.

Complete 10 to 12 repetitions.

HEAVY UP: If doing this exercise with only your body weight for resistance isn't sufficiently challenging, use medium or large dumbbells for added resistance.

CHANGE IT UP: Extend your arms in front of you so that they're level with your shoulders and parallel to the ground. Keep them in this position throughout the squat.

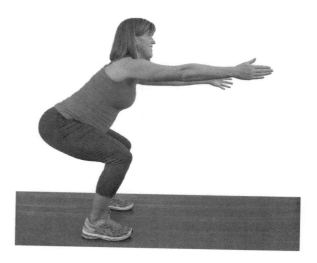

COMMON FAULTS: Don't allow your knees to cave inward or the arches of your feet to collapse. Keep your shins vertical to avoid placing shear forces on the soft tissues of the knee joint.

OVERHEAD SQUAT

Overhead squats can help correct anterior pelvic tilt (a common movement compensation during pregnancy), improve shoulder mobility, increase leg strength, and improve core strength. Due to decreased balance and possible sensitivity in your joints, you don't need to lower your thighs so that they're parallel with the floor. Stop before you feel discomfort.

STARTING POSITION: Stand in a braced neutral position with your feet significantly wider than shoulder-width apart, knees aligned over your ankles, and toes and knees turned out. Extend your arms overhead and out to the side slightly, as if forming a "Y," while keeping them in line with your ears. Don't allow your ribs to flare, meaning don't expand your ribcage and elevate your chest to compensate for limited shoulder mobility.

1. Hinge from your hips, lowering them toward the floor as you bend your knees. Push outward through your knees and keep the arches of your feet from collapsing. Keep your arms extended and in line with your ears throughout the move. Your trunk will tilt forward, but your spine should remain in a braced neutral position, maintaining adequate space for your baby.

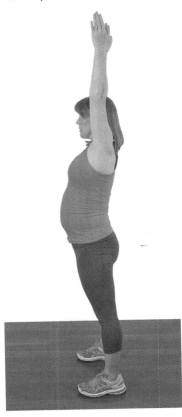

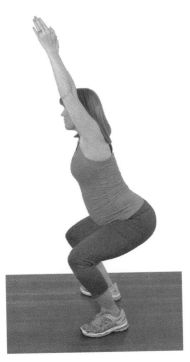

Press through your heels as you straighten your legs and rise to the starting position.

Complete 8 repetitions.

WALKING LUNGE

The pregnancy hormone relaxin increases flexibility and range of motion, particularly for exercises like lunges. While clinical research hasn't found any harm from this effect in exercise, be careful not to overdo it. Choose to exercise within the range of motion you had before pregnancy.

STARTING POSITION: Stand in a braced neutral position with your feet hip-width apart and arms at your sides.

1. Step forward with your right foot, planting your heel and bending your right knee until your thigh is nearly parallel with the floor. Bend your left knee toward the ground. Most of your weight should be on your front leg. Pause at the bottom of the move.

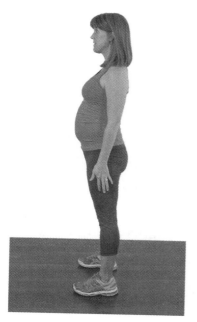

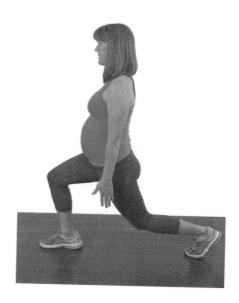

2. Push through the heel of your right leg and push off the floor with your left leg. Step forward with your left foot, planting the heel on the floor, and complete another lunge.

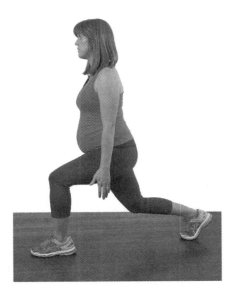

Repeat in one direction for a total of 10 to 12 lunges on each leg.

HEAVY UP: If doing this exercise with only your body weight for resistance isn't sufficiently challenging, use medium or large dumbbells for added resistance.

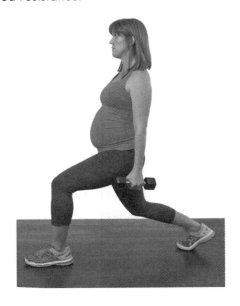

COMMON FAULTS: Place 90 percent of your weight on your front leg and lean forward somewhat, but don't allow your knee to extend past your toe.

STATIC LUNGE

If space is limited, opt for static lunges instead of walking lunges.

STARTING POSITION: Stand in a braced neutral position with your feet hip-width apart and arms at your sides.

1. Step forward with your right foot, planting your heel and bending your right knee until your thigh is nearly parallel with the floor. Bend your left knee toward the ground. Most of your weight should be on your front leg. Pause at the bottom of the move.

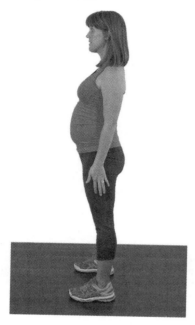

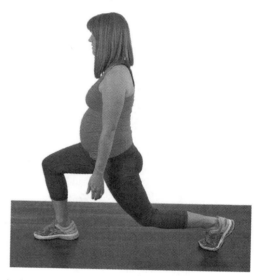

Push through the heel of your right leg and return to the starting position. Step forward with your left foot, planting the heel on the floor, and complete another lunge.

Complete 10 to 12 repetitions.

SIDE LUNGE

Put most of your weight into the bent leg and focus on bringing your hips toward the floor, not your chest.

STARTING POSITION: Stand in a braced neutral position with your feet hip-width apart and arms at your sides.

1. Step to the side with your right foot, planting your heel. Bend your right knee as you lower your hips toward the floor, keeping your left leg straight. Pause at the bottom of the move.

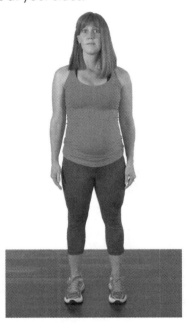

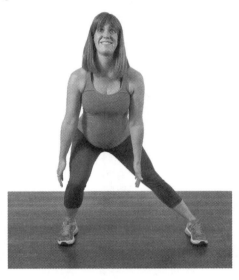

Push through the heel of your right leg and return to the starting position. Step to the side with your left foot, planting the heel on the floor, and complete another side lunge.

Complete 10 to 12 repetitions.

DEAD LIFT

Dead lifts are one of the best exercises for increasing hip mobility and leg strength, but they're also the easiest to do incorrectly. As you perform the exercise, think about reaching with your hips for an imaginary wall behind you and keeping your back perfectly flat. As your belly expands, widen your stance.

STARTING POSITION: Stand in a braced neutral position with your feet hip-width apart and arms at your sides.

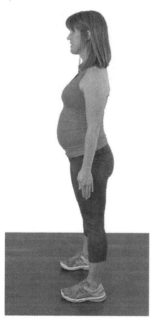

1. Hinge forward from your hips, maintaining a neutral spine and head position. Reach toward the floor until your torso is parallel with the ground. Allow your knees to bend slightly.

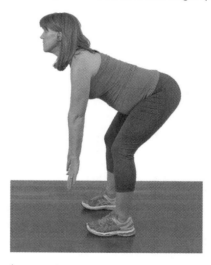

Rise to the starting position.

Complete 10 to 12 repetitions.

HEAVY UP: If doing this exercise with only your body weight for resistance isn't sufficiently challenging, use a barbell or two medium dumbbells for added resistance.

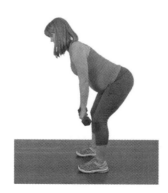

COMMON FAULTS: Avoid rounding your back or rounding your shoulders forward.

SHOULDER STRETCH

THE POSITION: Stand with your feet hip-width apart. Bring one arm across your body and hold it with the opposite arm for 30 seconds. Repeat on the other arm.

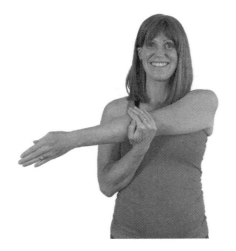

TRICEPS STRETCH

THE POSITION: Stand with your feet hip-width apart. Extend one arm overhead, bend it at the elbow, and reach it down toward your back. Hold the elbow with the opposite arm to deepen the stretch. Hold for 30 seconds. Repeat on the other arm.

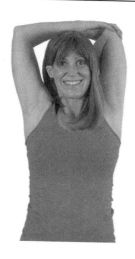

QUADRICEPS STRETCH

THE POSITION: Use a chair for balance and bring one heel toward your butt, holding onto the ankle with the same-side hand. Your heel should come toward your buttocks and not toward your outer thigh. Tuck your pelvis under to deepen the stretch. Hold for 30 seconds. Repeat on the other leg.

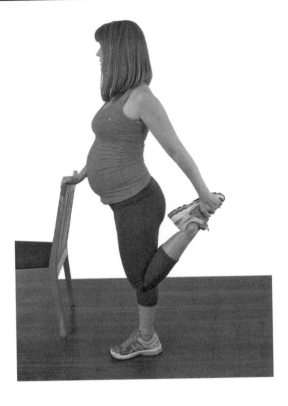

PSOAS LUNGE STRETCH

THE POSITION: Stand in a braced neutral position and step one foot forward slightly farther than a typical stride length. Distribute your weight evenly between both legs and lower the back knee toward the floor as you tuck your pelvis under. Gently rotate your torso slightly toward the front leg. Don't let your front leg go beyond 90 degrees. Hold for 30 seconds. Repeat on the other leg.

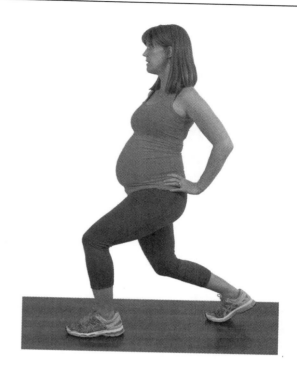

HAMSTRINGS STRETCH

THE POSITION: Stand with your feet hip-width apart and place one foot about 12 inches in front of you, with the heel on the floor, leg straight, and toe pointed upward. Bend the standing leg and reach toward your pointed toe with the same-side hand, grabbing it if you can. Hold for 30 seconds. Repeat on the other leg.

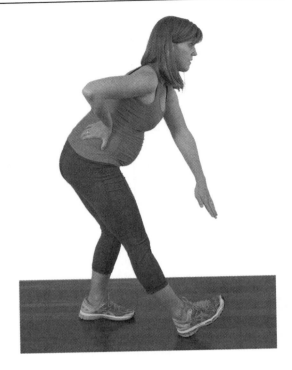

POSTPARTUM PREVENTION

Exercise in the hospital? Sure, it sounds crazy, but think of it like kegels, or the help you receive to develop healthy nursing posture. It's just a part of the recovery process.

These exercises, all of which can be done in the hospital, have been shown to reduce diastasis when performed in two sessions during the first 24 hours after birth. They're designed for women who've delivered vaginally without complications. If you've had a C-section or birth complications, wait until you receive your doctor's okay to begin these exercises.

The exercises are also helpful for women even years after delivery in that they begin to develop healthy breathing and movement patterns.

DIAPHRAGMATIC BREATHING

Your abdominal muscles assist the diaphragm, located at the base of your lungs, in exhalation.

STARTING POSITION: Lie on your back with your knees bent and feet flat on the bed or mat. Place your left hand just above your navel and your right hand over your upper chest.

1. Inhale slowly for 7 seconds and observe your left hand rising. Your right hand should remain still. Pause for 3 seconds.

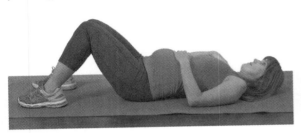

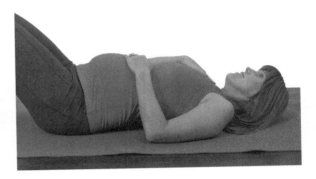

2. Exhale forcefully for 7 seconds and consciously contract your abdominal muscles, imagining bringing your right and left sides together. Repeat for 10 breathing cycles.

PELVIC TILT & CONTRACTION

This exercise engages your gluteal muscles and rectus abdominis to encourage posterior pelvic tilt. This motion is the opposite of anterior pelvic tilt, a movement compensation that most women develop during pregnancy to accommodate their changing body.

THE POSITION: Lie on your back with your knees bent and feet flat on the bed or mat.

Contract your gluteal muscles and hamstrings as you tuck your pelvis up and back. Imagine trying to thrust a Ping-Pong ball from your pelvis toward your head. Your hips should maintain contact with the bed or mat but shouldn't be bearing much weight. Hold the position for 20 seconds.

Relax for 10 seconds, then repeat for 10 contractions.

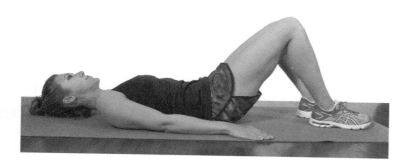

ABDOMINAL CONTRACTION

This exercise improves rectus abdominis tonicity, which is a state of normal tension and readiness to function in a muscle.

STARTING POSITION: Lie on your back with your knees bent and feet flat on the bed or mat. Place your hands behind your head to support it. Don't interlace your fingers; instead, stack your palms on one another.

1. Contract your rectus abdominis and elevate your head from the bed or mat just until the stomach muscles are engaged. Exhale for a count of 10 seconds as you hold the contraction. Release and relax for 5 seconds.

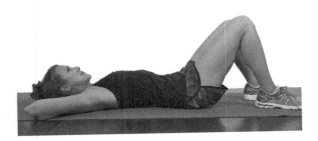

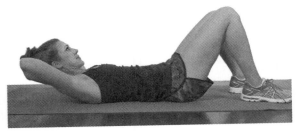

Complete 10 repetitions.

KEGELS

Kegels help restore pelvic floor strength and can be done from your hospital bed, while seated, or while standing.

THE POSITION: Lie on your back with your knees bent and feet flat on the bed or mat. Squeeze your pelvic floor muscles for 3 seconds and then release.

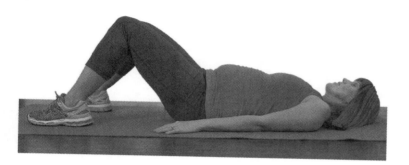

Part 3

TREATMENT

TREATMENT OVERVIEW

The treatment program I recommend is progressive and graded to your rate of recovery. It begins with Phase One, designed to activate your core muscles and help you develop proper movement and lifting patterns. Phase Two is designed to work your core stabilizing muscles and improve balance. Phase Three is designed to strengthen your whole body and provides the greatest core challenge. Each phase becomes more difficult and can be followed for as little as one week or up to four weeks. Use your own progress as your guide. Even if you're already fit, begin with Phase One and concentrate on doing the moves with proper form and without doming. If doming does occur, stay in that phase until you get stronger.

Each phase includes two workouts. The first incorporates total-body exercises, the second targeted core training. They can be performed independently for a 10-minute workout each day, or grouped together for a longer workout with a rest day in between. Focus your attention on performing each exercise with proper form.

These workouts can stand alone or be added to your existing exercise routine. It all depends on your goals and how much time you have to devote to physical activity. My goal was to provide the most effective exercises in the least amount of time.

Two exercises that can be done at any time will help heal the postural and pelvic floor effects of pregnancy: braced neutral spine and kegels. Add them to each workout in each phase, practicing daily.

BRACED NEUTRAL SPINE

The position is described in steps, but eventually you should be able to achieve braced neutral spine in one cohesive movement. It should be the foundation from which all movement originates, both in the gym and in daily life.

THE POSITION: Stand with your feet hip-width apart and arms at your sides.

Rotate your pelvis into a neutral position, neither tilted forward (arched lower back) nor tilted backward (rounded lower back). Your waistband should be level with the floor. Without moving your feet, contract your thighs as you rotate your hips out. Imagine that you're locking your feet in place.

Contract your abdominal muscles moderately, bracing as if someone is about to hit your stomach.

Stack your ribcage over your pelvis, allowing your ribs to descend and come together so that they're not splayed out. Lower your shoulders back and down and align your ears with your shoulders.

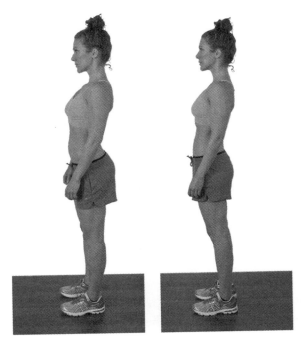

KEGELS

Kegels come in just behind braced neutral spine in order of importance for healing your postpartum body. They're easy to do and should be done daily. Although you may initially gain understanding of the contraction while urinating, they shouldn't be done repeatedly in that situation.

THE POSITION: Stand or sit with proper posture. Squeeze your pelvic floor muscles for 3 seconds and then release. Work up to holding the contraction for 7 seconds. Imagine that your pelvic floor is an elevator rising into your abdomen and practice by contracting it "upward" one level at a time.

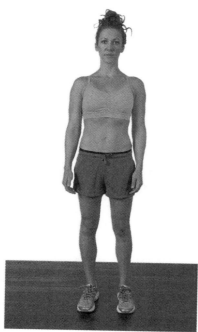

PHASE ONE—ACTIVATE

The initial phase of this program is designed to activate your core muscles and bring attention to proper movement and lifting patterns. No warm-up or cool-down is needed for this phase. For new moms, I include this graphic 🪇 and a brief description on how to do exercises with your baby where appropriate. Of course, you can do any exercise with your baby present, but some are fun to actually do with your baby.

WORKOUTS FOR PHASE ONE—ACTIVATE		
	EXERCISE	DURATION
Workout 1	Supine Thigh Adductor (page 57)	10 reps
	Glute Bridge (page 58)	3 reps
	Cat Pose (page 59)	10 reps
	Goblet Squat (page 60)	3 reps
Workout 2	Wall Plank (page 61)	3 reps
	Kneeling Hay Baler (page 62)	10 reps each leg
	Crunch (page 63)	10 reps
	Supine Alternating Bent-Knee Lift (page 64)	10 reps each leg

SUPINE THIGH ADDUCTOR

This exercise activates your abdominal, gluteal, and pelvic floor muscles through isometric contraction, meaning there's no visible movement through the joints. It's similar to the Pelvic Tilt & Contraction (page 49) in the Postpartum Prevention section, but this adds resistance.

STARTING POSITION: Lie on your back with your knees bent and feet flat on the mat. Place a pillow between your knees.

1. Tuck your pelvis under, gently squeeze your knees together, and contract your gluteal muscles. Hold for 10 seconds. While holding this position, contract and release your pelvic floor muscles.

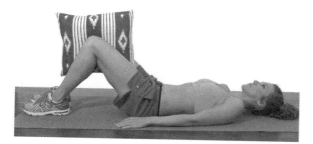

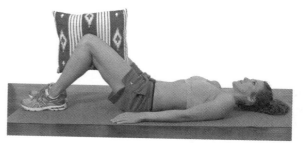

Return to the starting position and rest for 5 seconds.

Complete 10 repetitions.

CHANGE IT UP: The first time you perform this exercise, hold the pelvic floor contractions for 5 seconds and release for 5 seconds. As you gain control over your pelvic floor muscles, hold the contraction for the full 10 seconds.

 Allow your baby to rest on your chest during this exercise.

GLUTE BRIDGE

Continue building strength in your gluteal and pelvic floor muscles with this isometric exercise. As you hold the position, imagine tilting your pelvis up and back toward an imaginary point behind your head.

STARTING POSITION: Lie on your back with your knees bent and feet flat on the mat.

1. Tuck your pelvis under as you lift your hips off the floor, and contract your gluteal muscles and rectus abdominis.

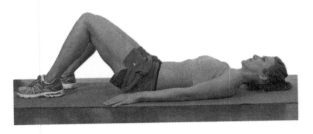

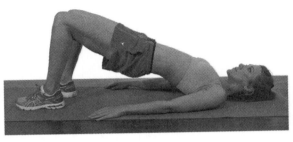

Hold the position for 20 seconds and then lower to the starting position.

Complete 3 repetitions.

 Allow your baby to rest on your chest during this exercise.

CAT POSE

This simple yoga pose helps correct anterior pelvic tilting and improves abdominal control and neutral spine. It's often paired with cow pose, but the spinal extension of cow pose can further stretch the linea alba if done through your full range of motion.

STARTING POSITION: Get on your hands and knees with a neutral spine and your eyes looking at the floor. Position your wrists directly beneath your shoulders and your knees directly beneath your hips.

1. Exhale and round your spine upward, allowing your head to descend toward the floor without forcing it.

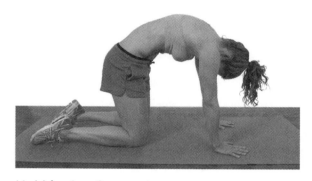

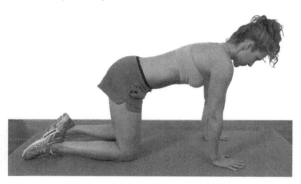

Hold for 1 to 2 seconds.

Inhale and return to the starting position.

Complete 10 repetitions.

Allow your baby to rest on the floor beneath you during this exercise. Open and close your eyes as you complete the move, as if playing peek-a-boo.

GOBLET SQUAT

Adding an isometric contraction to the bottom of the squat gives you an opportunity to consciously focus on contracting your abdominal muscles and maintaining a neutral spine. This exercise does wonders for your quadriceps, glutes, and abs.

STARTING POSITION: Stand in a braced neutral position with your feet slightly wider than shoulder-width apart, knees aligned over your ankles, and toes pointing forward or barely turned out. To increase resistance and improve stability, hold a dumbbell or another weighted object in front of you.

1. Lower your hips toward the floor as you bend your knees. Don't allow them to cave inward or the arches of your feet to collapse. Pause at the bottom of the move for 30 seconds, contracting your core muscles and maintaining a neutral spine.

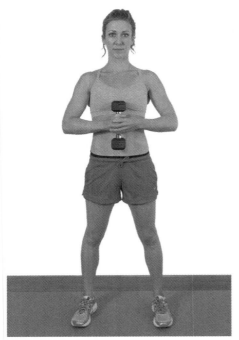

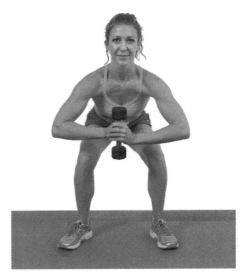

Press through your heels as you straighten your legs and rise to the starting position. Contract your gluteal muscles at the top of the move.

Complete 3 repetitions.

Instead of holding a dumbbell, hold your baby under her arms, having her face either toward you or away during this exercise.

WALL PLANK

Planks are an essential exercise for improving core and upper-body strength and learning how to hold neutral spine position under a challenging load. However, early in your recovery from diastasis, a horizontal plank performed on the floor may increase stretching of the linea alba. This modified plank looks easy, but it's valuable for developing core stability before you move on to traditional planks.

STARTING POSITION: Stand facing a wall with your arms extended and hands on the wall, shoulder-width apart.

1. Keeping your abdominals braced, bend your elbows and bring your chest toward the wall. Allow your heels to rise from the floor as needed.

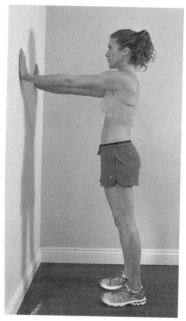

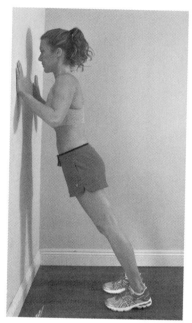

Hold the position a few inches from the wall for 10 seconds. Return to the starting position.

Complete 3 repetitions.

KNEELING HAY BALER

This exercise works the core and shoulders in the transverse, or rotational, plane of motion, which is where the majority of daily movement occurs (and also where the majority of injuries occur). Use your abdominal muscles to stabilize your spine throughout the movement.

STARTING POSITION: Get into a kneeling lunge position, with one leg bent and foot flat on the floor in front of you, and the opposite knee on the floor with your leg extended behind you. Hold a dumbbell or medicine ball in both hands near the hip of the rear leg.

1. Extend the weight toward the ceiling, crossing the midline of your body and twisting gently through your trunk until the weight is above the opposite shoulder.

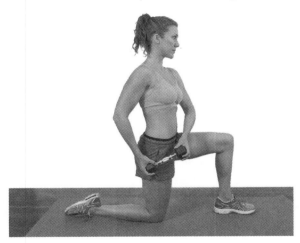
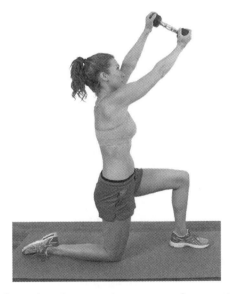

Slowly and with control, return to the starting position.

Repeat 10 times on one side and then repeat 10 times with the other leg leading.

Instead of using a dumbbell, hold your baby under his arms facing either toward you or away during this exercise. Unless you're very strong, this will be difficult if your baby weighs more than 10 pounds.

CRUNCH

When graded to your rate of recovery, crunches are an essential tool in rebuilding core strength and healing diastasis recti. The key is to avoid pushing past where you're comfortable and to avoid doming, which is when your lower abdomen protrudes at the most difficult part of the move. If this occurs, regress the exercise or perform the Abdominal Contraction (page 50) in the Postpartum Prevention section until you get stronger.

STARTING POSITION: Lie on your back with your knees bent and feet flat on the mat. Place your hands behind your head, stacking your palms on one another. Your elbows should be open without splaying your ribs. Maintain contact between the mat and your lower back.

1. Exhale, contracting your rectus abdominis, and elevate your head and shoulders from the mat toward the ceiling, maintaining contact between your lower back and the floor.

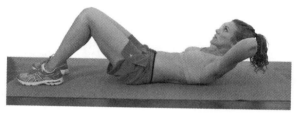

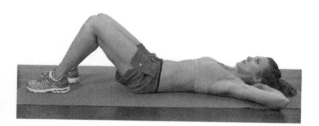

Inhale and slowly and with control, lower to the starting position.

Complete 10 repetitions.

SUPINE ALTERNATING BENT-KNEE LIFT

Before you progress to the straight-leg lifts popular in many abdominal routines and Pilates, do this version to build strength in your rectus abdominis and hip flexors.

STARTING POSITION: Lie on your back with your knees bent, legs lifted, and shins parallel to the mat. Allow your arms to rest at your sides.

1–2. Keeping the knee bent, lower one leg toward the floor and tap the mat with your toe. Repeat with the other leg.

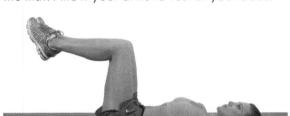

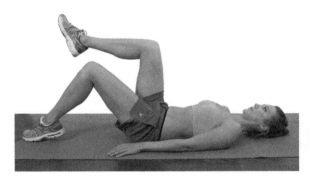

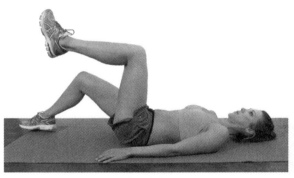

Alternate for a total of 20 repetitions.

Allow your baby to rest on your chest during this exercise.

PHASE TWO—BALANCE

This section is all about balance—balancing the muscles being worked and challenging them from different angles, as well as improving your balance and core stabilizing muscles. Some of the exercises in this section include a "finishing stretch." It's designed to stretch the muscles you just worked, which has been shown to improve strength and reduce tightness in the muscle. Plus, it just feels good!

WORKOUTS FOR PHASE TWO—BALANCE		
	EXERCISE	DURATION
Workout 1	Side-Lying Clamshell (page 66)	25 reps each side
	Glute Bridge with Leg Extension (page 67)	30 seconds each leg
	Extended Cat Pose (page 68)	10 reps each side
	Overhead Squat (page 69)	8 reps
	Walking Lunge with Chop (page 70)	10–12 reps each leg
Workout 2	Dead Bug (page 71)	10 reps
	Kneeling Psoas Stretch (page 72)	30 seconds each side
	Modified Plank (page 73)	10 seconds
	Reverse Crunch (page 74)	10 reps each side
	Oblique Twist (page 75)	10 reps each side
	Modified Side Plank (page 76)	30 seconds each side

SIDE-LYING CLAMSHELL

The first exercise in Phase One targeted the adductor muscles of your legs, which are located on the inner thigh and work to bring your legs toward your body. Your abductor muscles, located on the outer thigh, do the opposite, moving your legs away from your body.

STARTING POSITION: Lie on your side with your lower elbow bent and hand supporting your head. Stack your hips and knees on top of one another and bend your knees so that they're slightly in front of you. Your top arm can be placed on your hip, or you can place your palm on the floor in front of you. For added resistance, loop an exercise band around your legs just above your knees.

1. Keeping your heels together, lift the top knee until it points toward the ceiling.

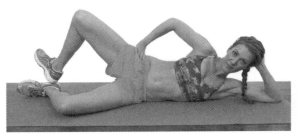

Slowly and with control, lower it to the starting position.

Complete 25 repetitions on each side.

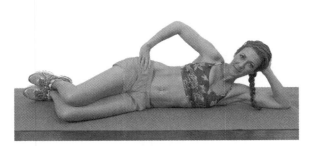

GLUTE BRIDGE WITH LEG EXTENSION

Increase the challenge of a basic glute bridge with this isometric contraction. It strengthens your core and gluteal muscles, and improves core stability.

STARTING POSITION: Lie on your back with your knees bent and feet flat on the mat.

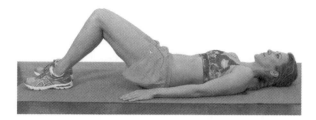

1. Tuck your pelvis under as you lift your hips off the floor and contract your gluteal muscles and rectus abdominis. Extend one leg so that both thighs are parallel. The leg on the floor is the working leg.

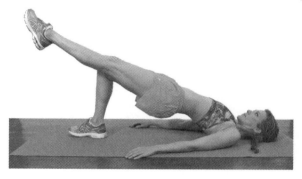

Hold the position for 30 seconds then lower to the starting position.

Repeat with the opposite leg.

FINISHING STRETCH: Sit on the floor with legs extended and reach forward to touch your toes. Hold the stretch for 20 to 30 seconds.

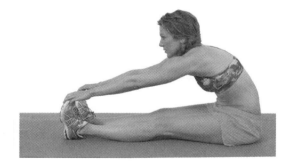

EXTENDED CAT POSE

This exercise improves core stability and balance while strengthening your gluteal and spinal erector muscles.

STARTING POSITION: Get onto your hands and knees with a neutral spine and your eyes facing the floor. Position your wrists directly beneath your shoulders and your knees directly beneath your hips.

1. Keeping your hips square and your spine in a neutral position, extend your left arm forward to shoulder level while you extend your right leg behind you. Your ribs should be level with your hips. Hold the position for 5 seconds.

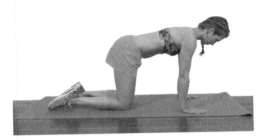

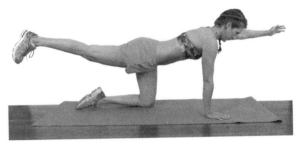

Return to the starting position.

Complete 10 repetitions and then switch sides.

FINISHING STRETCH: Perform child's pose by sitting back on your heels and extending your arms in front of you on the floor, allowing your head, chest, and abdomen to rest on the floor.

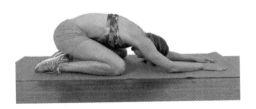

OVERHEAD SQUAT

Rarely does an exercise look so easy and feel as challenging as the overhead squat. The exercise is used by fitness professionals to assess a range of movement compensations and muscle imbalances. Learning to do this exercise correctly can help correct anterior pelvic tilt, improve shoulder mobility, increase leg strength, and improve core strength.

STARTING POSITION: Stand in a braced neutral position with your feet significantly wider than shoulder-width apart, knees aligned over your ankles, and toes and knees turned out. Extend your arms overhead and out to the sides slightly, as if forming a "Y," while keeping them in line with your ears throughout the move. Don't allow your ribs to flare.

1. Hinge from your hips as you bend your knees, lowering your hips toward the floor. Do not let your thighs go beyond parallel with the floor. This will be difficult initially. Push outward through your knees and keep the arches of your feet from collapsing. Your trunk will tilt forward slightly, but your spine should remain in a braced neutral position.

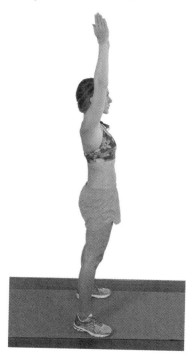

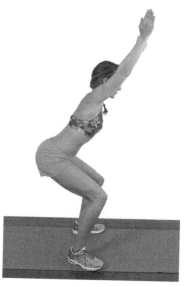

Press through your heels as you straighten your legs and rise to the starting position.

Complete 8 repetitions.

WALKING LUNGE WITH CHOP

Walking lunges work your legs and challenge your balance. Work in the transverse plane of motion as well by adding a twist.

STARTING POSITION: Stand in a braced neutral position with your feet hip-width apart. Hold a dumbbell or medicine ball in both hands and extend it overhead.

1. Step forward with your right foot, planting your heel and bending your right knee until your thigh is nearly parallel with the floor. Bend your left knee toward the ground. Most of your weight should be on your front leg. Simultaneously, lower the weight toward the hip of the back leg. Pause at the bottom of the move.

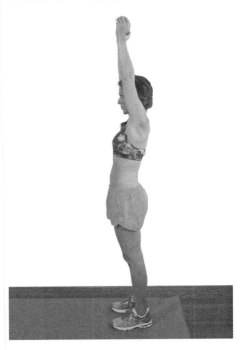

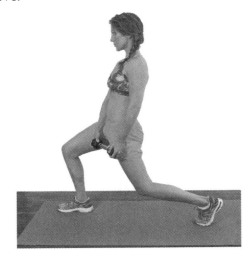

While lifting the weight overhead again, push through the heel of your right leg and push off the floor with your left leg.

Now step forward with your right foot, planting the heel on the floor and complete another lunge, this time rotating the weight to the opposite side.

Complete 10 to 12 lunges on each leg, 20 to 24 repetitions total.

DEAD BUG

This exercise is similar to the extended cat pose (page 68) but is done on your back to further challenge your abdominal muscles and improve shoulder mobility. Dead bug, coupled with the psoas stretch that follows, are essential exercises for correcting anterior pelvic tilt, which will improve the appearance of your stomach.

STARTING POSITION: Lie on your back with your legs extended over your hips, knees bent, shins parallel with the floor, and arms extended toward the ceiling over your shoulders.

1. Maintaining contact between the floor and your lower back, extend your right leg and left arm toward the floor. Keep your ribs from flaring.

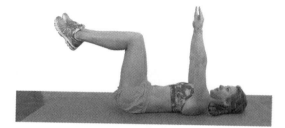

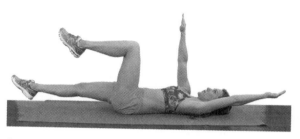

Return to the starting position and repeat with the left leg and right arm.

Complete 10 repetitions.

KNEELING PSOAS STRETCH

Part of correcting anterior pelvic tilt involves loosening tight hip flexors. This is a basic hip flexor stretch and specifically targets the psoas.

STARTING POSITION: Kneel in a shallow lunge position with the front knee bent, toe pointed forward, and back foot on the floor. Both legs should be bent 90 degrees.

1. Tuck your pelvis under and rotate your torso slightly toward the front knee.

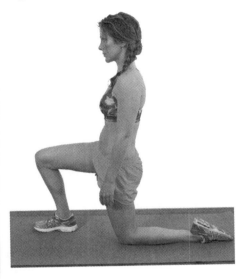

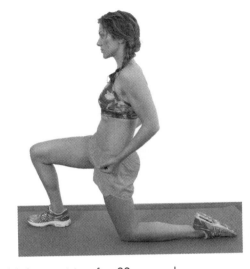

Hold the position for 30 seconds.

Repeat on the opposite side.

MODIFIED PLANK

Plank exercises challenge your core strength. Keep your gluteal muscles tight and your pelvis tucked under to protect your lower back. As soon as your stomach sags or you lose the correct form, stop the exercise. As you get stronger, work up from holding the plank for 10 seconds to 30 seconds.

STARTING POSITION: Lie on your stomach with your hands on the floor beneath your chest.

1. Contracting your abdominal and gluteal muscles and keeping your knees on the floor, press the floor away with your hands. Your neck should remain in alignment with your spine.

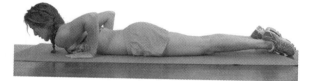

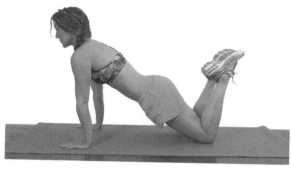

Hold the position for 10 seconds.

Rest and repeat for another 10 seconds.

REVERSE CRUNCH

The reverse crunch is one of the exercises used in the study mentioned on page 6 that evaluated the effects of exercise on diastasis recti. Women began performing this exercise two days after childbirth.

STARTING POSITION: Lie on your back with your legs extended over your hips, keeping your knees bent, shins parallel with the floor, and arms resting on the floor. Your lower back should be touching the floor.

1. Use your abdominal muscles to elevate your hips and draw your knees toward your chest.

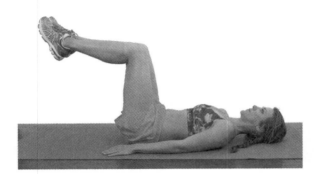

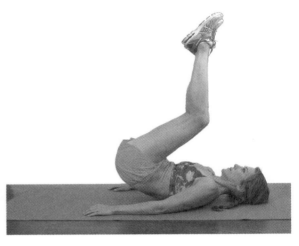

Slowly and with control, lower to the starting position.

Complete 20 repetitions.

OBLIQUE TWIST

This exercise strengthens the oblique muscles, which are positioned on your sides near your rib cage. They're involved in lateral (sideways) flexion and trunk rotation.

STARTING POSITION: Lie on your back on a mat with your knees bent and feet flat on the floor. Place your hands behind your head, stacking your palms on one another. Your elbows should be open without splaying your ribs. Maintain lower back contact with the mat.

1. Keeping your elbows open, elevate your right shoulder off the mat and twist toward your left knee.

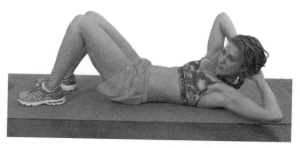

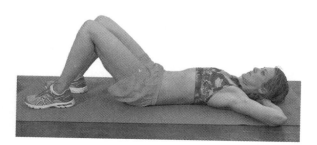

Lower and repeat on the opposite side, bringing your left shoulder off the mat and twisting toward your right knee.

Complete 20 repetitions.

MODIFIED SIDE PLANK

This exercise also strengthens the oblique muscles with an isometric contraction.

STARTING POSITION: Lie on one side with your forearm on the floor beneath your shoulder and your hips stacked over one another. Place your top hand on your hip.

1. Keeping your knees on the floor, lift your hips off the mat so that your body forms a straight line from your shoulders to your knees.

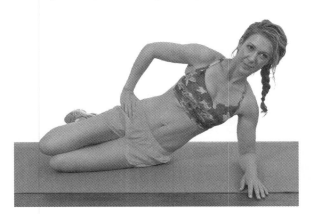
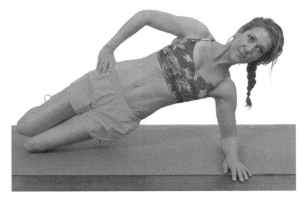

Contract your core to hold the position for 30 seconds.

Repeat on the opposite side.

PHASE THREE— STRENGTHEN

The exercises in Phase Three are more challenging than the previous two phases and work to strengthen your core muscles while protecting your diastasis from further stretching.

Because this section is all about strength, you should perform each exercise until you reach muscle failure (the point at which you cannot physically complete another repetition) or you can no longer complete the move with proper form, whichever comes first. Reaching muscle failure is what produces strength adaptations.

WORKOUTS FOR PHASE THREE—STRENGTHEN

	EXERCISE	DURATION
Workout 1	Push-Up (page 79)	as many as possible with good form
	Concentration Curl (page 80)	as many as possible with good form
	Arnold Press (page 81)	as many as possible with good form
	Wall Squat (page 82)	30–60 seconds
	Stability Ball Bridge & Curl (page 83)	as many as possible with good form
Workout 2	Plank (page 84)	minimum 60 seconds
	Side Plank (page 85)	60 seconds
	Alternating Straight-Leg Lift (page 86)	10 reps each side
	Reverse Oblique Twist (page 87)	10 reps each side
	Stability Ball Leg Lift (page 88)	10 reps

PUSH-UP

This total-body exercise strengthens your core, gluteal muscles, shoulders, and chest. Work up to performing the exercise on your toes, but don't advance the move unless your form is perfect.

STARTING POSITION: Lie on your stomach on the floor, keeping your elbows bent, your hands on the floor beneath your shoulders, and your toes on the floor. Contracting your core, press off the floor with your hands until your arms are extended and your body forms a straight line between your shoulders and your ankles. Your neck should remain in alignment with your spine.

1. Bend at your elbows and lower your chest toward the floor until your upper arms are level with your torso.

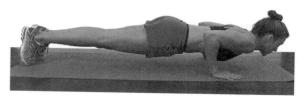

Complete as many repetitions as you can with good form.

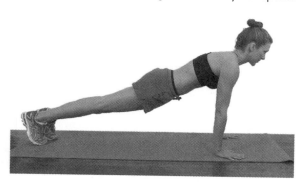

CONCENTRATION CURL

Carrying most newborns is easy enough, but as babies grow heavier and stronger, carrying them becomes increasingly challenging. Strengthen your arms for the task.

STARTING POSITION: Sit on the edge of a bench or chair with your feet wide and a heavy dumbbell in one hand, bracing your elbow on your inner thigh.

1. Curl the dumbbell, bringing it across your chest.

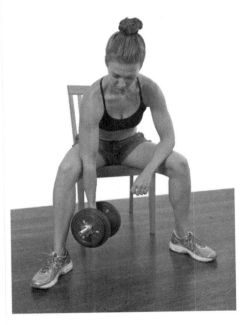

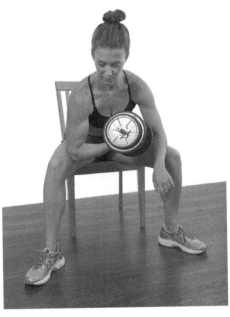

Slowly and with control, lower the dumbbell toward the floor.

Complete as many repetitions as you can with good form, and then repeat on the other side.

ARNOLD PRESS

This total-body exercise strengthens your shoulders, chest, and back.

STARTING POSITION: Stand in braced neutral spine position with a heavy dumbbell in each hand, palms facing your body and weights at your shoulders.

1. Press up, rotating the weights so that your palms face forward.

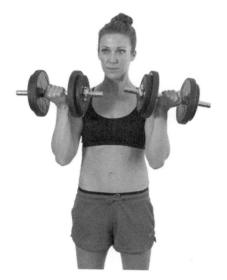

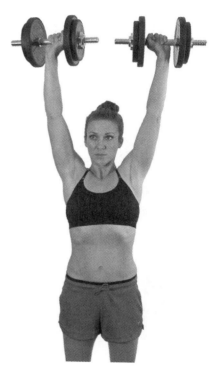

Slowly and with control, lower the weight back to starting position, rotating your palms inward again.

Complete as many repetitions as you can with good form.

WALL SQUAT

Traditional squats require a slightly forward position to maintain balance. Wall squats allow you to position your body weight farther back to target your quadriceps in a long isometric contraction.

THE POSITION: Stand with your back against a wall and your feet hip-width apart. Walk your feet away from the wall and lower your hips toward the floor. When your thighs are parallel with the floor, hold the position for 30 seconds, or as long as you can maintain the position with proper form, and then rise to the starting position.

CHANGE IT UP: To increase the challenge, extend one leg so that it's nearly parallel with the floor.

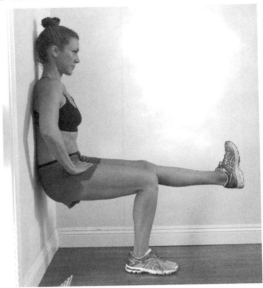

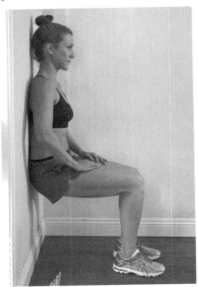

STABILITY BALL BRIDGE & CURL

This exercise works your hamstrings and challenges core stability.

STARTING POSITION: Lie on your back on a mat with your knees bent slightly and heels positioned on a stability ball. Elevate your hips into a bridge position, forming a straight line from your shoulders to your knees.

1. Bring your heels toward your butt, rolling the ball toward you and contracting your hamstrings.

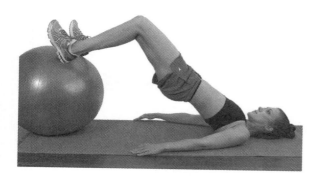

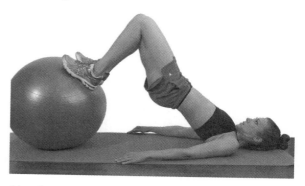

Slowly and with control, extend your legs and roll the ball away from you.

Complete as many repetitions as you can with good form.

PLANK

Perform planks on your hands and toes. To increase the challenge, reduce the angle of the plank by performing it on your forearms instead.

STARTING POSITION: Lie on your stomach on the floor with your elbows bent and your hands on the floor underneath your chest.

1. Contracting your core, press off the floor with your hands until your arms are extended and your body forms a straight line between your shoulders and your ankles. Your neck should remain in alignment with your spine.

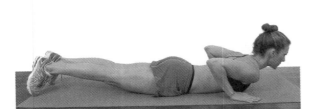

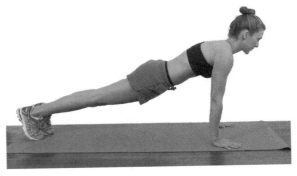

Hold the position for 60 seconds or until you reach muscle failure.

SIDE PLANK

Think about reaching your hips toward the ceiling as you perform this move. To regress the exercise, keep the supporting arm straight with your palm on the floor.

STARTING POSITION: Lie on one side with your forearm on the floor beneath your shoulder, and your feet and your hips stacked over one another. Extend your top arm toward the ceiling or place your hand on your hip.

1. Keeping your feet flexed and stacked, lift your hips off the mat so that your body forms a straight line from your shoulders to your feet.

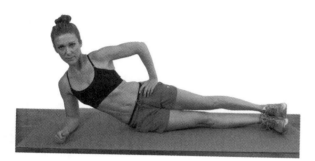

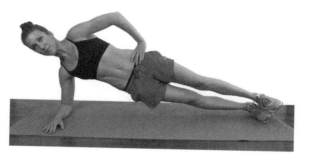

Contract your core to hold the position for 60 seconds or as long as you can maintain the position with proper form and then repeat on the other side.

ALTERNATING STRAIGHT-LEG LIFT

Resist the temptation to use your hip flexors to lift your legs and contract your rectus abdominis to complete the move. Initially perform the exercise with alternating legs and work up to doing the move with both legs at the same time. However, always regress the move if you notice doming in your stomach.

STARTING POSITION: Lie on your back on a mat with your legs extended and arms resting at your sides. Your lower back should be touching the mat.

1. Keeping both legs straight, raise one leg until your toe points toward the ceiling. Continue bringing the leg toward your chest and reach toward your ankle with both hands, allowing your shoulders to come off the mat slightly.

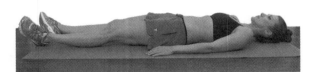

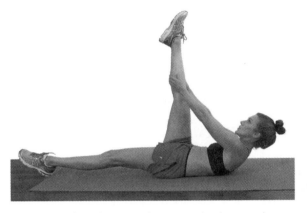

Slowly and with control, return the leg to the mat and repeat with the other leg.

Complete as many repetitions as you can until you reach muscle failure or can no longer perform the move with proper form.

REVERSE OBLIQUE TWIST

Similar to the reverse crunch, this exercise targets your rectus abdominis and obliques from a slightly different angle.

STARTING POSITION: Lie on your back with your knees bent, feet flat on the floor. Place your hands behind your head, stacking one on top of the other.

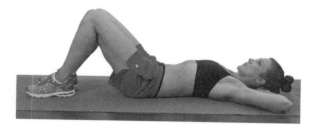

1. Contracting your abdominal muscles to lift your hips from the floor, twist through your abdomen to bring your knees toward one side of your body as you elevate the elbow and shoulder of that side toward your knees.

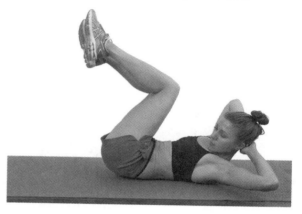

Lower and repeat, twisting to the opposite side.

Complete as many repetitions as you can until you reach muscle failure or can no longer perform the move with proper form.

STABILITY BALL LEG LIFT

If you don't have a stability ball, you can position a pillow between your feet or simply use your legs for resistance.

STARTING POSITION: Sit on a mat with your knees bent, toes on the floor, and your hands positioned slightly behind your hips. Hold a stability ball between your feet and maintain a braced neutral spine as you lean back on your hips slightly. Elevate your feet about six inches from the mat.

1. Extend your legs until they're straight and the ball is elevated. Your body should form a "V" shape.

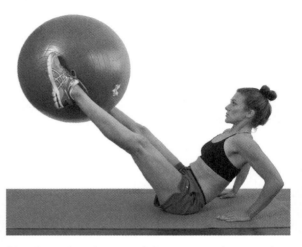

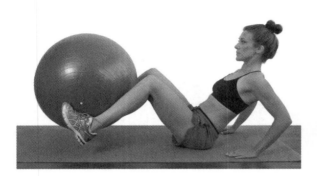

Slowly and with control, lower your legs to the starting position.

Complete as many repetitions as you can until you reach muscle failure or can no longer perform the move with proper form.

WEIGHT LOSS

The majority of clients I work with as a personal trainer want to lose weight, so I've devoted my training practice to the science of weight loss. I love helping people demystify the endless and often conflicting information on the topic so they can find freedom from being overweight, chronic dieting, and perpetual frustration.

In this chapter, I'll discuss research-based nutrition principles that will help you achieve sustainable weight loss without hunger or deprivation. I'll also cover the types of exercise that have been shown to contribute to weight loss.

A wide variety of approaches to weight loss can and do work, despite the claims of exclusivity made by so many popular diets. Research indicates that successful weight loss programs incorporate many if not all of the following strategies:

- Restrict total energy intake.

- Ensure adequate protein intake.

- Ensure plenty of non-starchy vegetables.

- Limit or eliminate processed foods.

- Limit or eliminate carbohydrates in the form of refined grains and sugar.

- Hydrate with water, not caloric beverages.

- Exercise with purpose.

In fact, simply adopting even one of these strategies can help you lose weight. Ultimately, the approach that yields sustainable weight loss with the least amount of hunger or stress is the best. Healthy habits should be something you can embrace as a lifestyle, not something you suffer through for a few days or weeks just to achieve temporary results.

Whether you've piled on pounds year after year, tried and failed at many diets, or continue to experience feelings of food addiction, give yourself permission to let go of the guilt and shame. They aren't doing you any favors. Learn to love yourself right where you're at and let your healthy choices emerge from that place of kindness toward yourself.

1. RESTRICT ENERGY INTAKE. Research indicates that modest calorie restriction can be successful at generating weight loss. It can be achieved through calorie counting, portion control, points systems, or any other method of reducing the amount of energy you consume (e.g., stopping a meal when you're 80 percent full, using smaller plates, etc.).

One pound of body fat is roughly equivalent to 3,500 calories. Hence, a deficit of about 350 calories per day through food intake restriction could theoretically generate one pound of fat loss in 10 days. Additionally, if you're breastfeeding, you'll burn 300 calories or more per day.[1] However, weight loss is more complex than a "calories in, calories out" equation. Where those calories come from affects how your body responds to the calorie deficit.

2. ENSURE ADEQUATE PROTEIN INTAKE. Dietary protein has a few things going for it when it comes to weight loss. First, it's satiating, meaning it makes you feel satisfied after a meal and for hours afterward. In fact, research evaluating the effects of protein on the brain finds that it doesn't stimulate appetite the same way carbohydrate and fat do. Second, some of the calories in protein are lost in the energy required to digest it. Finally, protein doesn't elevate blood glucose levels and insulin production to the same extent that carbohydrates (especially refined carbs) do. Protein is also purported to have muscle-sparing effects, meaning you'll replace muscle that's metabolized via the caloric deficit.

Protein should comprise 10 to 30 percent of your daily calories. It can come from plant or animal sources. However, protein from animal sources is more bioavailable, meaning more of it's absorbed and synthesized by your body. So if you're a vegetarian or vegan, you may want to slightly increase the amount of protein you aim for each day.

3. ENJOY PLENTY OF NON-STARCHY VEGETABLES. Vegetables are low in calories but rich in fiber, water, vitamins, minerals, antioxidants, and phytochemicals, meaning they'll support your weight-loss goals and your overall health. If you're accustomed to eating canned or frozen vegetables, branch out and try fresh, seasonal vegetables and new preparation methods. My favorite

---

1 According to the American College of Obstetrics and Gynecology, "Moderate weight reduction while nursing is safe and doesn't compromise neonatal weight gain."

ways to enjoy vegetables are oven-roasted or completely raw. Aim for four to five servings of vegetables each day.

4. LIMIT OR ELIMINATE PROCESSED FOODS. The slogan "betcha can't eat just one" could be applied to most processed foods (think breakfast cereals and frozen pizza, not bagged salads) because they override natural hunger and satiety mechanisms, so you eat more than you need to. Most processed foods are also bereft of nutritional value, meaning they supply plentiful calories, typically in the form of fat and sugar, but little fiber, protein, vitamins, or minerals. So you may feel full temporarily, but within an hour or two you'll feel sluggish and hungry again. This is a particularly challenging scenario in the early postpartum period, when sleep deprivation and the constant demands of a newborn predispose you to look for instant energy in the form of processed foods and make it difficult to prepare healthy meals.

Fortunately, there are many prepared foods sold in health food stores and the nutrition aisle of supermarkets that rival the healthy foods you might make at home. Think rotisserie chicken, pre-chopped vegetables, and pre-cooked brown rice. Once-weekly meal preparation and even meal delivery services are other options for keeping processed foods off the menu.

5. LIMIT OR ELIMINATE CARBOHYDRATES IN THE FORM OF REFINED GRAINS AND SUGAR. When you consume carbohydrates, your blood glucose rises and your pancreas releases insulin, which transports glucose to your cells. Some of the glucose is stored as glycogen in your muscles and liver, and some of it's stored as triglycerides in the liver and as body fat. The higher the rise in blood glucose, either by way of total glycemic load (how many carbs you consume) or glycemic index (how quickly the glucose enters your bloodstream), the more will be stored as body fat, particularly if your muscle glycogen stores are full.

Insulin doesn't stop there. It also suppresses hormone-sensitive lipase, which breaks down triglycerides into fatty acids. To put it plainly, insulin prevents your body from converting stored body fat into useable energy. Clearly, limiting sugar and simple carbohydrates is essential for weight loss.

Sugar and sugar substitutes are the worst offenders. High-fructose corn syrup, honey, maple syrup, agave, and, of course, white and brown sugar all have at least four grams of sugar per teaspoon.[2] Whether they're labeled organic, locally grown, raw, evaporated, or with any other health halo, sugars all have a similar effect on blood glucose and insulin production.

---

2 Non-caloric sugar substitutes are just as bad as the real thing. While they don't contain any sugar or carbohydrate, they trigger the release of insulin.

Simple carbohydrates such as white rice, potatoes, wheat flour, and gluten-free flours have a surprisingly similar effect as refined sugar, with some of the glucose hitting your bloodstream just as quickly. And because we tend to consume them in larger quantities, the total glycemic load is often higher.

However, not all carbohydrates produce this effect so severely, especially if you're active. Choose complex carbohydrates such as vegetables, sweet potatoes, quinoa, brown rice, lentils, beans, and fruit. These have a lesser effect on insulin production and will offer a steady stream of energy, improve your mood, quicken recovery from workouts, and help preserve muscle during weight loss.

6. HYDRATE WITH WATER, NOT CALORIC BEVERAGES. Proper hydration has numerous positive health effects, including supporting weight loss. First, drinking enough water prevents you from confusing thirst with hunger. Second, it has a small thermogenic effect, meaning you burn calories as you warm the liquid to body temperature. Finally, proper hydration has the inverse effect of keeping you from retaining water, so, although it doesn't equal fat loss, it does create a slimmer physique.

Caloric beverages, on the other hand, stimulate insulin production and are dehydrating if they contain caffeine or alcohol.

Aim for at least 96 ounces of water daily. I like to fill a three-quart pitcher in the morning and finish it by dinner time. Infusing water with a few slices of fruit and herbs can help you reach your daily goal. Sparkling water is another option, although it may cause some air to fill the stomach and cause a bloated appearance.

7. EXERCISE WITH PURPOSE. Exercise may or may not support your weight-loss goals. It all depends on why you exercise and how you define it. Make sure when you exercise, you do it deliberately. You should also strive to sit less.

Exercise should never be about burning calories. Think about it this way: It takes a few moments to consume 150 calories, say, in the form of a chocolate chip cookie, but takes as many as 20 minutes of jogging to burn it off. The math just doesn't support exercise as a method of calorie burning, especially because it may increase appetite or increase license to indulge in more calories than were burned.

Here are several better reasons to exercise for weight loss. First, it can improve insulin sensitivity, meaning your body has to release less insulin to handle blood glucose. Less insulin equals less fat storage. Second, it can improve fat oxidation during exercise so that, as your aerobic capacity increases, your ability to burn fat during exercise also increases. Additionally, exercise depletes muscle glycogen stores so that when you consume carbohydrates, the influx of glucose has a place to go. Exercise can also increase lean body mass, which has modest positive effects on your metabolism.

How you define exercise influences its ability to generate weight loss. There are three essential components to exercising for weight loss—high-intensity interval training, intense resistance training, and moderate cardiovascular exercise. Also, non-exercise activity thermogenesis (NEAT) refers to the amount of energy burned doing daily tasks such as standing, folding laundry, and walking up stairs, and is as effective at generating weight loss as more deliberate methods. In fact, not getting enough NEAT throughout the day is worse than skipping the gym altogether.

For weight-loss clients, I recommend a total of 4 to 6 hours of exercise a week, or 45 to 60 minutes on most days, with rest days at least once a week.

High-intensity interval training (HIIT) has been shown to specifically utilize stored belly fat and improve aerobic capacity and preferential fat burning, so it should comprise a total of 30 minutes of your weekly training program—a little goes a long way. I've included a brief HIIT workout at the end of this chapter. The exercises can be interspersed throughout other workouts or done independently as a quick and effective weight-loss workout.

Resistance training is the most effective when it provides actual resistance. That sounds redundant, but for the number of three-pound neoprene dumbbells still gracing women's fitness magazines and workout classes, it apparently still needs to be said. If you can lift it 30 times while dancing, that's endurance training (which has its own value), not resistance training. Instead, choose weights that are heavy enough that you can perform no more than 15 repetitions. The last reps should be difficult to impossible to complete.

Ultimately, diet still plays a more significant role than exercise in weight loss. This is good news, especially for newly postpartum moms who want to lose weight but don't have the time or desire to spend countless hours in the gym. A 2015 systematic review of research on the effect of weight management interventions among pregnant and postpartum women observed that dietary interventions were five times more effective than physical activity on weight loss. Other studies have observed similar effects: exercise confers modest weight-loss benefits, but nutrition is key. An article published in the *British Medical Journal* put it plainly: "You cannot outrun a bad diet."

FLEXIBLE DIETING

If you've already adopted these strategies but still have a few pounds to lose or have specific body composition goals in mind, consider flexible dieting, a method I recommend to many of my clients. It involves careful tracking of calories and macronutrients but allows freedom for a variety of food with the caveat, "if it fits your macros," or IIFYM.

Although tracking every macronutrient sounds like a lot of work, research shows that people who log their calories lose 57 percent more weight than "intuitive eaters." Treat it like a math game, and approach it without fear or stress. Do your best each day and know that every day is a learning opportunity.

CALCULATE TOTAL DAILY ENERGY EXPENDITURE

Begin by calculating your basal metabolic rate, BMR, with the following equation:

$$
\begin{aligned}
& 655.1 \\
+ \ & (4.35 \times \underline{\quad} \text{ weight in pounds}) \\
+ \ & (4.7 \ \times \underline{\quad} \text{ height in inches}) \\
- \ & (4.7 \ \times \underline{\quad} \text{ age in years}) \\
\hline
= \ & \text{BMR}
\end{aligned}
$$

Multiply your BMR by your activity level to determine your total daily energy expenditure, TDEE.[3]

Sedentary to light exercise, 1 hour per week: 1.1

Moderate exercise, 2 to 3 hours per week: 1.2

Intense exercise, 4 or more hours per week: 1.35

$$\text{BMR} \times \text{Activity Level} = \text{TDEE}$$

Subtract 20 percent from your TDEE to determine the number of calories you should consume each day.

$$\text{TDEE} - 20\% = \text{calories for weight loss}$$

---

3 These numbers are slightly lower than most activity calculators because others simply overestimate how many calories you're actually burning.

For example, a 32-year-old woman who weighs 145 pounds, is 5'4" tall, and exercises 2 hours each week would've made the following calculations:

$$655.1 + (4.35 \times 145 = 631) + (4.7 \times 64 = 301) - (4.7 \times 32 = 150) = 1437 \text{ BMR}$$

$$1437 \times 1.2 = 1724 \text{ TDEE}$$

$$1724 \text{ TDEE} - 20\% = 1380 \text{ calories}$$

CALCULATE MACRONUTRIENTS

Divide the calories needed for weight loss between the three macronutrients: protein, fat, and carbohydrate. Protein and carbohydrate contain 4 calories per gram and fat contains 9 calories per gram.

To calculate how much protein you need, multiply your current body weight in pounds by .8.

Example: 145 x .8 = 116 grams protein.[4]

To calculate how much fat you need, multiply your current body weight in pounds by .2 or .3. (Personally, I feel better using the .3 calculation.)

Example: 145 x .3 = 43.5 grams fat

116 grams of protein x 4 calories per gram = 464 calories

43.5 grams of fat x 9 calories per gram = 391.5 calories

Once you calculate your protein and fat needs, the remaining calories can come from carbohydrate and should include at least 25 grams of fiber.

1380 calories – 464 – 391.5 = 524 calories, 131 grams carbohydrate

How you break up those calories into macronutrients isn't an exact science. Ultimately, you have to listen to your body.

Once you know your macros, use them to plan meals and snacks. Foods can be whatever you enjoy and whatever fits your personal preferences. Hence, paleo dieters, vegans, those with food restrictions, and even picky eaters can put flexible dieting principles to work. Use a pen and paper and a calculator, or opt for a free online calorie tracker, such as MyFitnessPal.

---

4 Your body can't metabolize large amounts of protein at one time, so space it throughout the day, aiming for about 30 grams at each meal and 5 to 10 grams in snacks, depending on your individual protein needs.

HIIT WORKOUT

I developed this workout to get your heart pumping during five intense intervals (one set of each exercise) followed by equivalent active recovery periods. The entire workout can be completed in 15 minutes, including warming up and cooling down. Do all exercises as hard as you can for 30 seconds, then do an active recovery for 30 seconds (such as gentle marching in place, toe taps, or shallow kicks) before moving on to the next exercise.

It's especially important to warm up before commencing a high-intensity interval workout. You can warm up with a light jog on a treadmill or outside, or do the four warm-up exercises I detail below for 3 to 5 minutes.

When cooling down, allow your heart rate to come down naturally by doing active recovery movements such as gentle marching, toe taps, and shallow kicks. Then proceed with the four static stretches I've detailed below.

Unless you've remained very active throughout your pregnancy, wait to commence this workout until you're at least six weeks postpartum, or until your doctor gives you the okay. If at any time you feel dizzy, faint, or can't catch your breath, stop immediately and consult your doctor.

This set of exercises is designed to be scalable to your fitness level. You should decide what feels appropriately challenging based on your fitness level and how rested you are. I often begin with the advanced version of the move and regress to the beginner version if I cannot complete the reps with proper form. Here's an example of how burpees can be scaled from an advanced version to a beginner version.

ADVANCED: For full burpees, squat and jump back into plank position, perform a push-up from the toes, jump forward to plank, and perform another squat jump with an overhead reach at the top of the move.

BEGINNER: To regress burpees, walk your feet back into plank position, do a push-up from your knees, walk your feet toward your hands, and simply stand upright to complete the move.

HIIT WORKOUT

	EXERCISE	DURATION
Warm-Up	Marching (page 98)	60 seconds
Warm-Up	Shallow Squat (page 99)	60 seconds
Warm-Up	Side-to-Side Toe Touch (page 100)	60 seconds
Warm-Up	High Knee Lift (page 101)	60 seconds
Workout 1	Mountain Climber (page 102)	30 seconds
Workout 1	Jumping Jack (page 103)	30 seconds
Workout 1	Burpee (page 104)	30 seconds
Workout 1	Side Skate (page 106)	30 seconds
Workout 1	Squat Jump (page 107)	30 seconds
Cool-Down	Calf Stretch (page 108)	30 seconds, each leg
Cool-Down	Kneeling Wall Stretch (page 108)	30 seconds
Cool-Down	Runner's Pose (page 109)	30 seconds, each leg
Cool-Down	Hip Stretch (page 109)	30 seconds, each leg

MARCHING

STARTING POSITION: Stand with your feet hip-width apart and your arms at your sides.

1. March in place, allowing your arms to swing naturally by your sides.

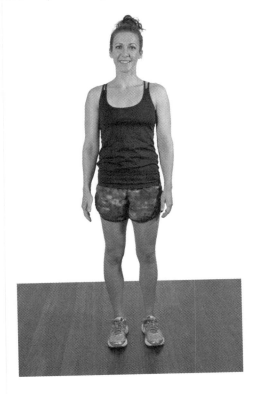

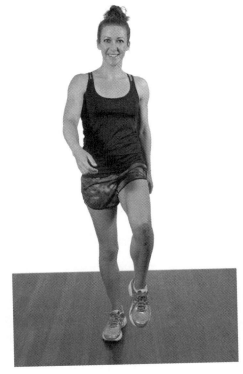

Continue for 60 seconds.

SHALLOW SQUAT

STARTING POSITION: Stand with your feet hip-width apart and your hands on your hips.

1. Keeping your toes and knees pointed forward, lower your hips toward the floor into a shallow squat.

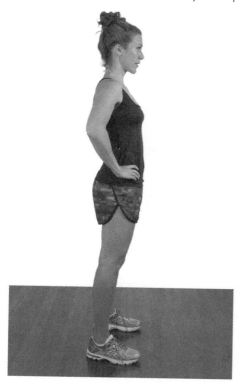

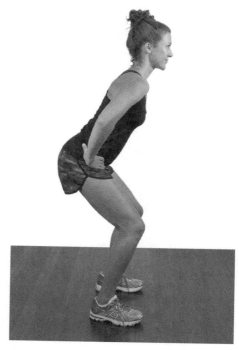

Press through your heels to stand.

Repeat for 60 seconds.

SIDE-TO-SIDE TOE TOUCH

STARTING POSITION: Stand with your feet hip-width apart and your arms at your sides.

1. While you tap one foot to the side, sweep your arms up until they're extended overhead. Think jumping jacks without the jump.

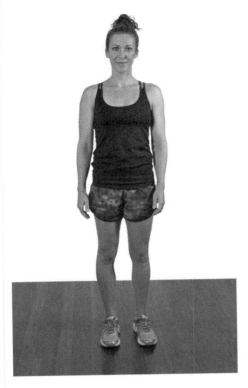

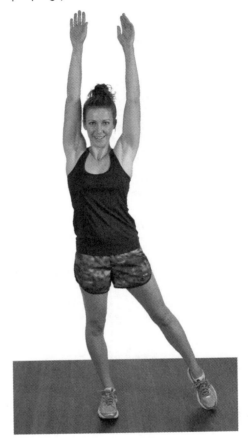

Lower your arms to your sides as you tap the opposite foot to the side.

Repeat for 60 seconds.

HIGH KNEE LIFT

STARTING POSITION: Stand with your feet hip-width apart and your arms at your sides.

1. Lift one knee until your thigh is parallel with the floor and pat it gently with your hands.

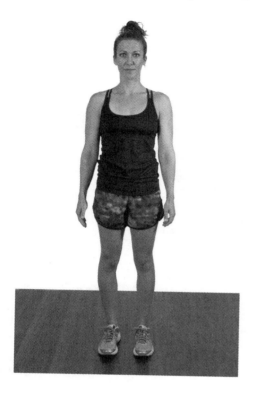

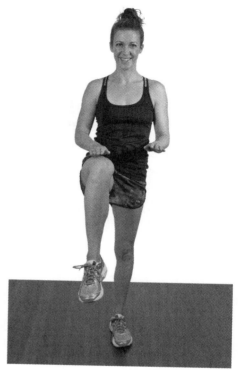

Lower, and lift the other knee.

Repeat for 60 seconds.

MOUNTAIN CLIMBER

Get your heart pumping and challenge your upper body and core with this exercise. For a greater challenge, jump each leg forward instead of stepping forward.

STARTING POSITION: Get into plank position with your arms straight, hands directly beneath your shoulders, and toes on the floor.

1–2. Bring one knee in toward your chest, touching the toe to the floor beneath your torso. Return it to the starting position and bring the opposite leg forward.

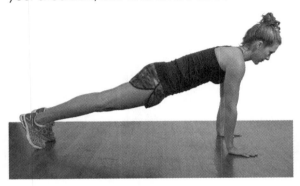

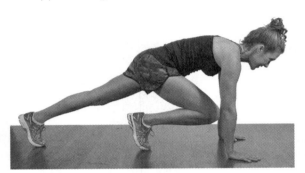

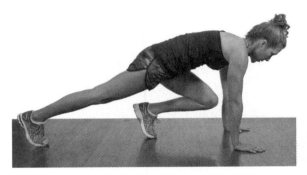

Continue for the duration of the interval.

JUMPING JACK

We all know this gym class staple, but don't underestimate its power to get your heart racing. Keep your armpits facing forward through the movement to protect your shoulder joints. If the jumping jack becomes too challenging, simply step your feet out to the side as in the warm-up, but do it as quickly as you can.

STARTING POSITION: Stand with your feet hip-width apart and your arms at your sides.

1. Jump your feet outward while you raise your hands overhead. Jump your feet back together and return your hands to your sides.

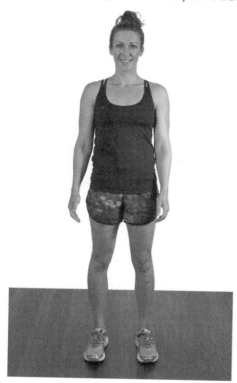

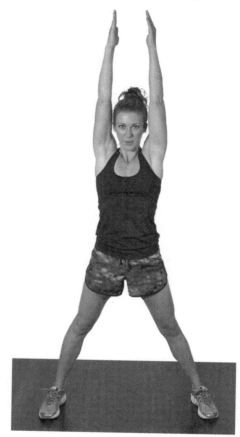

Repeat for the duration of the interval.

BURPEE

Burpees are one of the most intense body-weight exercises and build both stamina and strength. There's even a T-shirt that reads, "Burpees don't like you, either." Embrace the challenge, and you'll get stronger and shed pounds.

STARTING POSITION: Stand with your feet hip-width apart and arms at your sides.

1. Squat deeply and place your hands on the floor on either side of your feet.

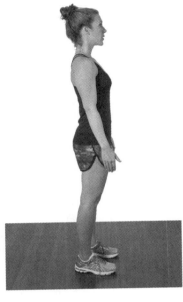

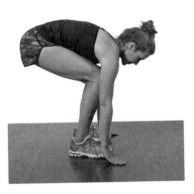

2. Jump or step your feet back into a plank position.

3. Do a push-up, or simply remain in plank position.

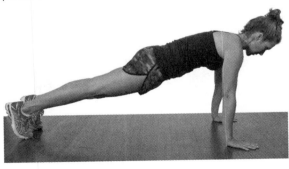

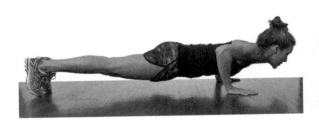

4. Jump or step your feet forward so they're between your hands.

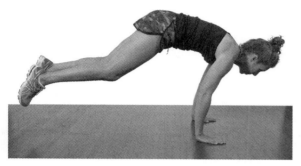

5. Stand up and extend your arms overhead, adding a jump for greater challenge.

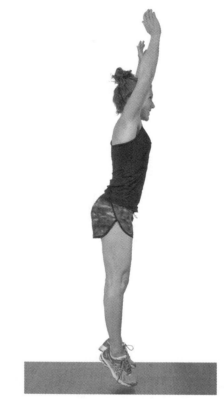

Repeat for the duration of the interval.

SIDE SKATE

Our daily movements are in all planes of motion, and our workouts should be, too. This move is in the frontal and transverse planes, involving side-to-side and twisting motions.

STARTING POSITION: Stand with your feet hip-width apart and your arms at your sides.

1. Leap or step to your right side with your right foot and tap your left foot behind you in a shallow curtsey. Reach your left arm toward your right foot.

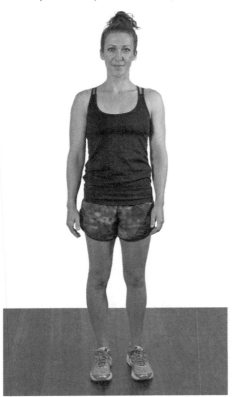

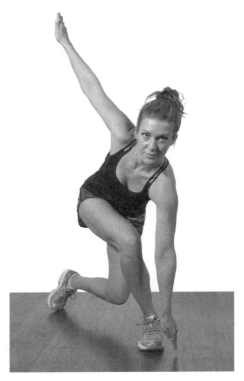

Repeat on the opposite side, leaping or stepping to your left with your left foot, tapping your right foot behind you, and reaching your right arm toward your left foot.

Repeat for the duration of the interval.

SQUAT JUMP

Make sure to keep your abdominals braced and your pelvis tucked under without arching your back during squat jumps to prevent urinary leakage, which is a problem for many women after giving birth.

STARTING POSITION: Stand with your feet slightly wider than hip-width apart and your arms at your sides. Lower your hips toward the floor, bending your knees and reaching your hands toward the sides of each foot until your thighs are parallel to the ground.

1. Jump as high as you can, reaching your arms overhead.

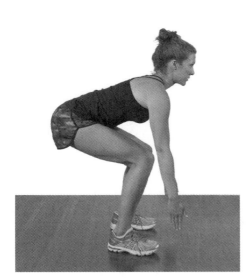

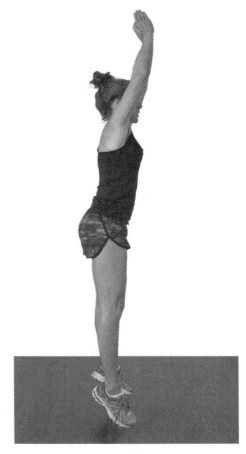

Repeat for the duration of the interval.

REGRESSION: If a standard squat jump is too challenging, keep your squat shallow.

CALF STRETCH

THE POSITION: Stand facing a wall and step one foot behind you. Press through your heel to feel a stretch in your calf. Hold for 30 seconds. Repeat with the other leg.

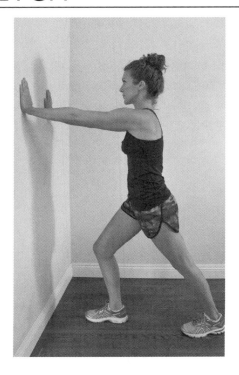

KNEELING WALL STRETCH

THE POSITION: Assume a low lunge position, with your back knee resting on a towel or cushion about 8 inches from a wall, and the top of your foot elevated and pressing against the wall. Keeping your hips square, lean forward slightly. Hold for 30 seconds.

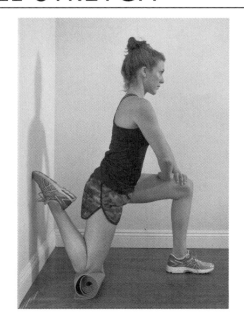

RUNNER'S POSE

THE POSITION: Step into a long lunge so that your front thigh is parallel with the floor. Reach toward the floor with your fingertips. Hold for 30 seconds. Repeat with the other leg.

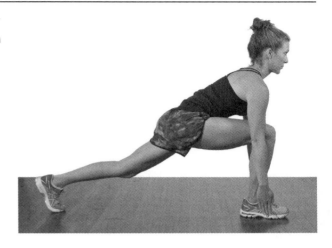

HIP STRETCH

THE POSITION: Lie on your back with your knees bent, feet flat on the floor. Place one ankle over the thigh of the opposite leg and pull this leg toward your chest, keeping the opposite knee turned out. Hold for 30 seconds. Repeat with the other leg.

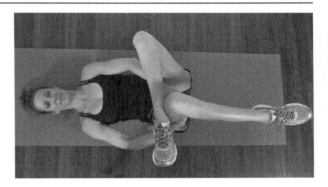

REFERENCES

Akram, J., and S. H. Matzen. "Rectus abdominis diastasis." *Journal of Plastic Surgery and Hand Surgery* (June 2014). doi:10.3109/2000656X.2013.859145.

Artal, R. and M. O'Toole. "Guidelines of the American College of Obstetricians and Gynecologists for exercise during pregnancy and the postpartum period." *British Journal of Sports Medicine* 37 (2003). doi:10.1136/bjsm.37.1.6.

Aune, D., et al. "Physical activity and the risk of gestational diabetes mellitus: a systematic review and dose-response meta-analysis of epidemiological studies." *European Journal of Epidemiology*. (August 2016). doi: 10.1007/s10654-016-0176-0.

Bellido, L. J. "Totally endoscopic surgery on diastasis recti associated with midline hernias. The advantages of a minimally invasive approach. Prospective cohort study." *Hernia* 19, no. 3 (June 2015) 493-501. doi: 10.1007/s10029-014-1300-2.

Belluz, J. and J. Zarracina. "Why you shouldn't exercise to lose weight." Show Me The Evidence. *Vox*. Accessed September 2016. http://www.vox.com/2016/4/28/11518804/weight-loss-exercise -myth-burn-calories.

Benjamin, D. R., et al. "Effects of exercise on diastasis of the rectus abdominis muscle in the antenatal and postnatal periods: a systematic review." *Physiotherapy* 100, no. 1. (March 2014) 1–8. doi: 10.1016/j.physio.2013.08.005.

Bø, K., et al. "Pelvic floor muscle function, pelvic floor dysfunction and diastasis recti abdominis: prospective cohort study." *Neurourology and Urodynamics* (March 2016). doi: 10.1002/nau.23005.

Bowman, K. *Diastasis Recti: The Whole-Body Solution to Abdominal Weakness and Separation.* Propriometrics Press, 2015.

Brauman, D. "Diastasis recti: clinical anatomy." *Plastic and Reconstructive Surgery* 122, no. 5 (November 2008) 1564–9. doi: 10.1097/PRS.0b013e3181882493

Cheesborough, J. E. and G. A. Dumanian. "Simultaneous prosthetic mesh abdominal wall reconstruction with abdominoplasty for ventral hernia and severe rectus diastasis repairs." *Plastic and Reconstructive Surgery* 135, no. 1 (January 2015) 267–76. doi: 10.1097/PRS.0000000000000840.

Chiarello, C. M. and J. A. McAuley. "Concurrent validity of calipers and ultrasound imaging to measure interrecti distance." *Journal of Orthopaedic and Sports Physical Therapy* 43, no. 7 (2013) 495-503. doi: 10.2519/jospt.2013.4449.

Chiarello, C. M., et al. "The effects of an exercise program on diastasis recti abdominis in pregnant women." *Journal of Women's Health Physical Therapy* 29, no. 1 (Spring 2005) 11–16. doi: 10.1097/01274882-200529010-00003.

Cholewicki, J., et al. "Can increased intra-abdominal pressure in humans be decoupled from trunk muscle co-contraction during steady state isometric exertions?" *European Journal of Applied Physiology* 81, no. 2 (June 2002) 127–33. doi: 10.1007/s00421-002-0598-0.

Cleveland Clinic. "Diaphragmatic breathing." Accessed August 2016. http://my.clevelandclinic.org/health/diseases_conditions/hic_Understanding_COPD/hic_Pulmonary_Rehabilitation_Is_it_for_You/hic_Diaphragmatic_Breathing.

Coleman, T. J. "Effects of walking speeds and carrying techniques on intra-abdominal pressure in women." *International Urogynecology Journal* 26, no. 7 (July 2015) 967–74. doi: 10.1007/s00192-014-2593-5.

El-Mekawy, H., et al. "Effect of abdominal exercises versus abdominal supporting belt on postpartum abdominal efficiency and rectus separation." World Academy of Science, Engineering and Technology, International Science Index 73, *International Journal of Medical, Health, Biomedical, Bioengineering and Pharmaceutical Engineering* 7, no. 1 (2013) 75–79.

Esser, K. "How to fix your anterior pelvic tilt." Accessed August 2016. http://kaseyesser.com/blog-post/how-to-fix-your-anterior-pelvic-tilt-part-1.

Fernandes da Mota, P. G., et al. "Prevalence and risk factors of diastasis recti abdominis from late pregnancy to 6 months postpartum, and relationship with lumbo-pelvic pain." *Manual Therapy* 20, no. 1 (February 2015) 200–5. doi: 10.1016/j.math.2014.09.002.

Grenier, S. G. and S. M. McGill. "Quantification of lumbar stability by using 2 different abdominal activation strategies." *Archives of Physical Medicine and Rehabilitation* 88, no. 1 (January 2007) 54–62. doi: 10.1016/j.apmr.2006.10.014.

Haddow, G., et al. "Effectiveness of a pelvic floor muscle exercise program on urinary incontinence following childbirth." *International Journal of Evidence-Based Healthcare* 3, no. 5 (May 2005) 103–46. doi: 10.1111/j.1479-6988.2005.00023.x.

Keshwani, N. and L. McLean. "Ultrasound imaging in postpartum women with diastasis recti: intrarater between-session reliability." *The Journal of Orthopaedic and Sports Physical Therapy* 45, no. 9 (September 2015) 713–8. doi: 10.2519/jospt.2015.5879.

Krucik, G. Medical review, "What causes lordosis?" Healthline. Accessed July 2016. http://www.healthline.com/symptom/lordosis.

Lee, D. and P. W. Hodges. "Behavior of the linea alba during a curl-up task in diastasis rectus abdominis: an observational study." *Journal of Orthopaedic and Sports Physical Therapy* 46, no. 9 (July 2016) 580–9. doi: 10.2519/jospt.2016.6536.

Lee, D. G. "Stability, continence and breathing: the role of fascia following pregnancy and delivery." *Journal of Bodywork and Movement Therapies* 12, no. 4 (October 2008) 333–348. doi: http://dx.doi.org/10.1016/j.jbmt.2008.05.003.

Liaw, L. et al. "The relationships between inter-recti distance measured by ultrasound imaging and abdominal muscle function in postpartum women: a 6-month follow-up study." *Journal of Orthopaedic and Sports Physical Therapy* 41, no. 6 (2011) 435–443. doi: 10.2519/jospt.2011.3507.

MacDonald, C., "Mother and baby yoga is good for you." *The Practicing Midwife* 16, no. 5 (May 2013) 14, 16, 18. http://www.ncbi.nlm.nih.gov/pubmed/23789249.

Malhotra, A., et al. "It's time to bust the myth of physical inactivity and obesity: you cannot outrun a bad diet." *British Journal of Sports Medicine* 49, no 15 (August 2015) 967–8. doi:10.1136/bjsports-2015-094911.

Mesquita, L. A., et al. "Physiotherapy for reduction of diastasis of the recti abdominis muscles in the postpartum period." *Revisita Brasileira de Ginecologia e Obstetrcia* 21, no. 5 (June 1999). doi: 10.1590/s0100-72031999000500004.

Middlekauff, M. L., et al. "The impact of acute and chronic strenuous exercise on pelvic floor muscle strength and support in nulliparous healthy women." *American Journal of Obstetrics and Gynecology* 215, no. 3 (September 2016) 1–7. doi: 10.1016/j.ajog.2016.02.031.

Monash University. "The Monash University Low-FODMAP Diet." Accessed September 2016. http://www.med.monash.edu/cecs/gastro/fodmap/low-high.html.

Mota, P., et al. "The immediate effects on inter-rectus distance of abdominal crunch and drawing-in exercises during pregnancy and the postpartum period." *Journal of Orthopaedic and Sports Physical Therapy* 45, no. 10 (October 2015) 781–8. doi: 10.2519/jospt.2015.5459.

Move Forward Physical Therapy. "Physical Therapist's Guide to Diastasis Rectus Abdominis." Accessed April 6, 2016. http://www.moveforwardpt.com/symptomsconditionsdetail.aspx?cid=f8a7ad12-eadf-4f42-9537-e00a399c6a03.

Muktabhant, B., et al. "Diet or exercise, or both, for preventing excessive weight gain in pregnancy." *Cochrane Database System Review* 15, no. 6 (June 2015). doi: 10.1002/14651858.CD007145.pub3.

MuTuSystem. "Diastasis recti." Accessed February 2016. https://mutusystem.com/ diastasis-recti.

Nall, Rachel. "Hernia after c-section; What are the symptoms?" Healthline. Accessed August 2016. http://www.healthline.com/health/pregnancy/hernia-after-c-section#Occurrence3

Noakes, M., et al. "Effect of an energy-restricted, high-protein, low-fat diet relative to a conventional high-carbohydrate, low-fat diet on weight loss, body composition, nutritional status, and markers of cardiovascular health in obese women." *American Journal of Clinical Nutrition* 81, no. 6 (June 2005) 1298–1306. http://www.ncbi.nlm.nih.gov/pubmed/15941879.

Pascoal, A. G. et al. "Inter-rectus distance in postpartum women can be reduced by isometric contraction of abdominal muscles: a preliminary case-control study." *Physiotherapy* 100, no. 4 (December 2014) 344–8. doi: 10.1016/j.physio.2013.11.006.

Perales, M., et al. "Benefits of aerobic or resistance training during pregnancy on maternal health and perinatal outcomes: a systematic review." *Early Human Development* 94 (March 2016) 43–8. doi: 10.1016/j.earlhumdev.2016.01.004.

Riley, Meredith. *Why diastasis recti experts disagree and what this means for your postpartum belly.* Motherfigure, 2015.

Sancho, M. F., et al. "Abdominal exercises affect inter-rectus distance in postpartum women; a two-dimensional ultrasound study." *Physiotherapy* 101, no. 3 (September 2015) 286–91. doi: 10.1016/ j.physio.2015.04.004.

Sheppard, S. "The role of transversus abdominis in correction of gross divarication recti." *Manual Therapy* 1, no. 4 (September 1996) 214–216. doi: 10.1054.math.1996.0272.

Speck, James. "4 great exercises for correcting anterior pelvic tilt." Somastruct. Accessed July 2016. http://www.somastruct.com/4-great-exercises-for-correcting-anterior-pelvic-tilt.

Spencer, L., et al. "The effect of weight management interventions that include a diet component on weight-related outcomes in pregnant and postpartum women: a systematic review protocol." *JBI Database of Systematic Reviews and Implementation Reports* 13, no. 1 (January 2015) 88–98. doi: 10.11124/jbisrir-2015-1812.

Staelens, A. S., et al. "Intra-abdominal pressure measurements in term pregnancy and postpartum: an observational study." *PLoS One* 9, no. 8 (August 2014). doi: 10.1371/journal.pone.0104782.

Starrett, Kelly. *Becoming a Supple Leopard.* 2nd edition. Victory Belt Publishing: May 2015.

Stillerman, Elaine. "A common problem for new moms and professional athletes." *Massage Today.* Accessed September 2016. http://www.massagetoday.com/mpacms/mt/article.php?id=14465.

Tupler Technique. Accessed February 2016. http://diastasisrehab.com.

UCSF Medical Center. "Ventral hernia." Accessed August 2016. https://www.ucsfhealth.org/conditions/ventral_hernia.

WebMD. "Kegel exercises: topic overview." Women's Health. Accessed September 15, 2016. http://www.webmd.com/women/tc/kegel-exercises-topic-overview.

Willardson, Jeffrey M. ed. By NSCA. *Developing the Core*. Champaign, IL: Human Kinetics 2014.

Wong, Mark., "How to fix an anterior pelvic tilt." *Posture Direct*. Accessed August 2016. http://posturedirect.com/fix-anterior-pelvic-tilt.

INDEX

Abdominal Contraction, 50
Abdominal exercise, 15–16; "doming," 17
Abdominal muscles, 8
Abdominal protrusion, 10–11
Abdominal strength, reduced, 10
Activate (Phase 1), workouts, 53, 56–64
Age, and diastasis recti, 10
Alternating Straight-Leg Lift, 86
Antagonist (resisting) muscles, 15
Anterior pelvic tilt, and belly protrusion, 19
Arnold Press, 81

Balance (Phase 2), workouts, 53, 65–76
Beer belly (visceral fat), 20
Belly protrusion, 8–9, 10–11; other causes, 19–20
Biceps Curl, 30
Blood glucose, 91
Braced neutral spine position, 15, 54
Bridges, 58, 67, 83
Burpees, 96; exercise, 104–105

Calf Stretch, 108
Caliper test, 12
Calorie intake, 90, 92
Carbohydrates, 91
Cat Pose, 59

Cesarean section (C-section): hernias, 13; post-partum exercises, 47
Concentration Curl, 80
Cool-down stretches, 22, 108–109; and HIIT workouts, 96
Crunches, 16; exercise, 63, 74
Curls, 30, 31, 80, 83

Dead Bug, 71
Dead Lift, 41
Diaphragmatic Breathing, 48
Diastasis recti, 8–20; causes, 9–10; defined, 8; diagnostic criteria, 8–9; prevention/treatment, 13–19; risks, 12–13; symptoms, 10–11; test, 11–12; variations, illustrated, 9
Digestive problems, and belly protrusion, 19–20
"Doming," and abdominal exercise, 17
Drawing-in maneuver, 16

Exercises: postpartum, 14; prenatal, 13–14; prevention, 22–51; strength/flexibility, 24–26; to avoid, 14; treatment exercises, 53–88; weight loss, 92–109
Extended Cat Pose, 68
External oblique muscles, 8

Flexible dieting concept, 94
Front Kick & Punch, 27

Frontal Deltoid Raise, 28
Glute Bridge, 58
Glute Bridge with Leg Extension, 67
Goblet Squat, 60

Hammer Curl, 31
Hamstrings Stretch, 46
Hernias, 13
High Knee Lift, 26, 101
HIIT (high-intensity interval training), 93,
    96–109
Hip Stretch, 109
Hospital exercises, 47–51
Hydration, 92

Insulin, 91
Inter-rectus distance, 16
Internal oblique muscles, 8

Jumping Jack, 103

Kegels, 51, 55
Kneeling Hay Baler, 62
Kneeling Psoas Stretch, 72
Kneeling Wall Stretch, 108

Lat Row, 33
Lateral Deltoid Raise, 29
Linea alba, 8, 9
Low back pain, 12–13
Lunges, 37–38, 39, 40, 45, 70

Macronutrients, 94–95
Marching, 24, 98
Modified Plank, 73
Modified Side Plank, 76
Mountain Climber, 102
Movement, and diastasis recti, 14
Muscle failure, 77

Muscles, 8, 15
NEAT (non-exercise activity thermogenesis), 93
Nutrition, 18; and weight loss, 90–92

Oblique muscles, 8
Oblique Twist, 75
Overhead Squat, 36, 69

Pelvic floor disorders, 12
Pelvic Tilt & Contraction, 49
Phase 1 (activate) workouts, 53, 56–64; exercises,
    57–64; program, 56
Phase 2 (balance) workouts, 53, 65–76; exercises,
    66–76; program, 65
Phase 3 (strengthen) workouts, 53, 77–88;
    exercises, 79–88; program, 78
Plank (basic), 84
Planks, 61, 73, 76, 84, 85
Postpartum exercises, 14, 47–51
Postpartum support belts, 17–18
Posture, 15
Pregnancy, exercises, 22–46
Prenatal exercise, 13–14, 22–46
Prevention exercises: postpartum, 14, 47–51;
    pregnancy, 22–46
Processed foods, 91
Protein intake, 90
Psoas Lunge Stretch, 45
Push-Up, 79

Quadriceps Stretch, 44

Raises, 28, 29
Rectus abdominis muscles, 8
Relaxin (hormone), 37
Resistance training, 93
Reverse Crunch, 74
Reverse Oblique Twist, 87
Risks, and diastasis recti, 12–13

Runner's Pose, 109
Shallow Squat, 99
Shoulder Stretch, 42
Side Lunge, 40
Side-Lying Clamshell, 66
Side Plank, 85
Side Skate, 106
Side-to-Side Toe Touch, 100
Side Toe Touch & Arm Raise, 25
Squat (basic), 34–35
Squat Jump, 107
Squats, 34–35, 36, 60, 69, 82, 99, 107
Stability Ball Bridge & Curl, 83
Stability Ball Leg Lift, 88
Starrett, Kelly, 15
Static Lunge, 39
Strength/Flexibility Workout, 22–46; exercises,
    24–46; program, 23
Strength training, 14
Strengthen (Phase 3), workouts, 53, 77–88
Stretches and stretching, 22, 42–46, 72, 108–109
Sugar substitutes, 91
Supine Alternating Bent-Knee Lift, 64
Supine Thigh Adductor, 57
Support belts, 17–18
Surgery, and diastasis recti, 18–19
Synergist (helping) muscles, 15

TDEE (total daily energy expenditure), 94–95
Tests, for diastasis recti, 11–12
Transversus abdominis muscles, 8
Treatment exercises, 53–88; phase 1 (activate),
    56–64; phase 2 (balance), 65–76; phase 3
    (strengthen), 77–88
Triceps Dip, 32
Triceps Stretch, 43
Twists, 75, 87

Ultrasound imaging test, 12

Vegetables, 90–91
Vegetarians, and protein, 90
Ventral hernias, 13
Visceral fat, and belly protrusion, 20

Walking Lunge, 37–38
Walking Lunge with Chop, 70
Wall Plank, 61
Wall Squat, 82
Warm-ups, 22; and HIIT workouts, 96
Water, drinking, 92
Weight loss workout, 89–109; exercises, 98–109;
    overview, 96; program, 97
Weightlifting, and diastasis recti, 10
Workouts: strength/flexibility, 22–46; phase 1,
    53, 56–64; phase 2, 53, 65–76; phase 3, 53,
    77–88; weight loss, 96–109

ACKNOWLEDGMENTS

I'm so grateful to my family for their love and support, especially my kids Brad and Cole.

Thanks to my husband Rich, who did all of the photography for this book. As always, it's so fun to work with you.

Special thanks to model Meagan Stirling for modeling for the pregnancy exercise section of this book. I can't wait to meet your new little one!

Special thanks to the editorial team at Ulysses, particularly Casie Vogel, Claire Chun, and Shayna Keyles, for shaping the direction and quality of this book.

ABOUT THE AUTHOR

Pamela Ellgen is a certified personal trainer with the National Academy of Sports Medicine. She is the author of several books on cooking, nutrition, and fitness, including *Psoas Strength and Flexibility*, *Cast Iron Paleo*, and *The Microbiome Cookbook*. Her work has also been published in *Huffington Post*, LIVESTRONG, *Darling Magazine*, Peak Pilates, and Spinning.com. Pamela lives in Santa Barbara, California, with her husband, Rich, and their two sons. When she's not training clients on the beach or cooking healthy meals, she enjoys surfing and exploring the local farmer's market.